Surface and Living

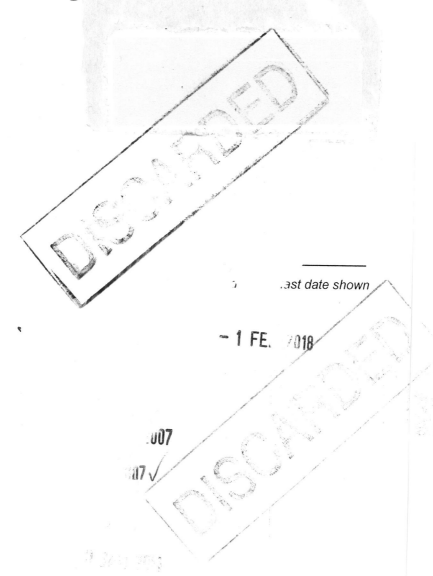

To Joan

For Mosby:

Senior Commissioning Editor: Sarena Wolfaard
Project Manager: Derek Robertson
Design Direction: Judith Wright

Surface and Living Anatomy

An Illustrated Guide for the Therapist

Gordon Joslin OStJ MCSP DipTP GradDip FCCAc
Tadley, Hampshire, UK

with

Raylene Collyer BA(MBK) HED
Teacher and Alternative Medicine Practitioner, London, UK

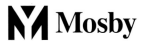 Mosby

MOSBY
An imprint of Elsevier Science Limited

First published 2002

ISBN 0 7234 3261 9

British Library Cataloguing in Publication Data
A catalogue record for this book is available from the British Library

Library of Congress Cataloging in Publication Data
A catalog record for this book is available from the Library of Congress

Note
Medical knowledge is constantly changing. As new information becomes available, changes in treatment, procedures, equipment and the use of drugs become necessary. The authors and the publishers have taken care to ensure that the information given in this text is accurate and up-to-date. However, readers are strongly advised to confirm that the information, especially with regard to drug usage, complies with the latest legislation and standards of practice.

The publisher's policy is to use **paper manufactured from sustainable forests**

Printed in China by RDC Group Limited

Contents

Preface

Many students studying complementary anatomy for the first time experience difficulty learning surface and living anatomy. The aim of this book and the accompanying CD-ROM is to provide access to a method of learning based on behavioural objectives. Each objective states in clear and unambiguous terms the performance to be demonstrated, the standard to be achieved and the conditions. The objectives are given in full on the CD-ROM and most are accompanied by colour images.

To achieve a standard of competence, students are required to progress through a series of logical steps or criteria by which anatomical structures are identified by palpation. These steps are listed with each objective.

The key to success in this step-by-step learning method is knowing where to start, and to progress in simple, clear and related steps to reach the desired standard of competence.

This book gives an insight into what can be achieved by using clear learning objectives and methods to achieve safe and competent standards of knowledge of surface and living anatomy.

Acknowledgements

Without the generous and unstinting support of friends and family this project could not have been conceived. My thanks to the following most patient, generous and long-suffering special people: Mrs Joan Murphy and family, Judy Gibbons and Lee Panter.

    Thanks are also due to Simon Murphy and Trevor Wing who provided the technical support and encouragement to purchase the equipment and learn computer skills.

Gordon Joslin, 2002

Bony Features of the Upper Limb

1. Spine of scapula
2. Clavicle
3. Apex of the coracoid process
4. Acromion process
5. Greater tubercle of humerus
6. Lesser tubercle of humerus
7. Medial epicondyle of humerus
8. Lateral epicondyle of humerus
9. Olecranon process of ulna
10. Head of ulna
11. Head of radius
12. Styloid process of radius
13. Styloid process of ulna
14. Dorsal tubercle of radius
15. Posterior border of shaft of ulna
16. Pisiform
17. Hamate
18. Trapezium
19. Scaphoid
20. Lunate

1. SPINE OF SCAPULA

There are two ways to achieve identification by palpation:

First method

1. Identify by palpation the spine of the **7th cervical vertebra** using the criteria contained in *Objective No 161*.
2. Count down from the tip of the **7th cervical vertebra**, identifying the tip of the **1st thoracic spinous process**, the tip of the **2nd thoracic spinous process** and the tip of the **3rd thoracic spinous process**.
3. Flexion of the cervical and upper thoracic areas of the vertebral column will help with identification.
4. Keep two fingertips in contact with the skin, one maintaining contact with a confirmed anatomical feature and the second fingertip identifying the next bony structure.
5. The **3rd thoracic spinous process** lies opposite the base of the **spine of scapula**.
6. The base of the **spine of scapula** is positioned approximately 5 cm from the midline at the level of the **3rd thoracic spinous process**.
7. Placing the tip of the index finger on the base of the **spine of scapula**, trace the prominent bony spine which feels like a ridge of bone, upwards and laterally to where it terminates as a flattened plateau of bone named the **acromion process** which forms the highest bony point of the **shoulder girdle**.
8. With the model in the anatomical position, ask the model to place the **dorsum** of the right hand, the **elbow joint** fully flexed, on the posterior aspect of the **thorax** in the midline between both scapulae.
9. The inferior angle of the scapula becomes visibly prominent and can be identified by palpation opposite the spinous process of the **7th thoracic vertebra**.
10. The vertebral border of the **scapula** can be clearly palpated to the base of the spine of scapula level with the spinous process of the 3rd thoracic vertebra.

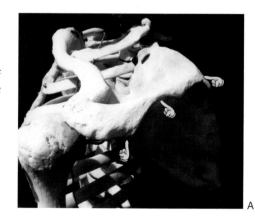

A

Second method

1. Ask the model to put the palmar surface of one hand on the upper fibres of the **trapezius muscle** (*Objective No 29*) of the opposite side.
2. The palmar surface of the fingertips should point downwards and be in contact with the **posterior surface of the thorax**.
3. A distinct bony ridge can be palpated just below the fingertips and moves when the **shoulder girdle** is moved.
4. Palpate this prominent bony ridge from its vertebral base upwards and outwards in a lateral direction to a flat subcutaneous bony area where it ends.
5. This flat subcutaneous bony area is the **acromion process** and is the highest bony point of the shoulder.
6. This prominent ridge running from medial to lateral, upwards and outwards is the **spine of scapula** which terminates in the **acromion process**.

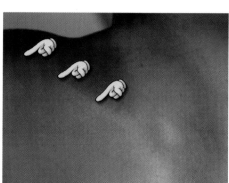

B

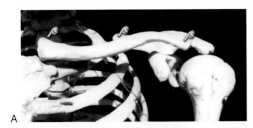

A

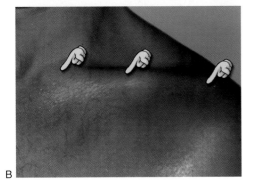

B

2. CLAVICLE

1. Palpate the **jugular notch** on the superior border of the **manubrium** on the **sternum** in the median plane.
2. Move the fingertip in a lateral direction to feel the raised and expanded **medial extremity of the clavicle**.
3. Keeping the fingertip on the **manubrium of the sternum** and raised extremity of the **clavicle**, ask the model to raise the shoulder point. The **sternoclavicular joint** can be identified where movement can be felt.
4. Palpate in a lateral direction from the expanded **medial extremity of the clavicle** along the **subcutaneous** and observable shaft of the clavicle to its junction with the **acromion process of the scapula**.
5. Place the tip of the palpating finger on the **acromion process of the scapula** pointing in a medial direction towards the **lateral extremity of the clavicle**. Keep the fingertip at 45° to the surface of the **acromion**.
6. Move the fingertip in a medial direction until a raised ridge is encountered showing the position of the **lateral extremity of the clavicle**.
7. Maintain the palpating finger on this feature and with the other hand grasp the model's **humerus** and apply gentle downward pressure.
8. Movement can be felt under the palpating finger at the joint line of the **acromioclavicular joint** which marks the junction between the **lateral extremity of the clavicle** and the **acromion process of the scapula**.

3. APEX OF THE CORACOID PROCESS

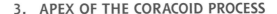

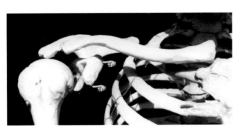

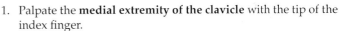

1. Palpate the **medial extremity of the clavicle** with the tip of the index finger.
2. Keep the tip of the middle finger in contact and parallel with the index finger.
3. Palpate the **shaft of the clavicle** with the index finger and move towards the **lateral extremity** with the middle finger inferior to the index finger.
4. At a point 2 cm inferior to the junction of the outer quarter of the shaft with the remaining three-quarters, a bony prominence can be felt underneath the **anterior fibres of the deltoid muscle** by the tip of the middle finger.
5. This prominent bony feature lying deep to the **anterior fibres of the deltoid** is the **apex of the coracoid process**.

4. ACROMION PROCESS

1. Follow the guidelines in criterion 1 to identify the **spine of scapula** (*Objective No 1*).
2. Palpate the **spine of scapula** and move in a lateral and superior direction towards the top of the shoulder.
3. About 2 cm from the top of the shoulder a sharp bony angle can be identified at the most lateral extremity of the spine of scapula. This bony feature is the **acromial angle**.

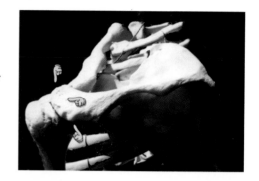

5. GREATER TUBERCLE OF HUMERUS

1. Identify the **acromion process** (*Objective No 4*).
2. Palpate the posterior acromial angle.
3. Move the palpating fingers forward along the prominent lateral edge of the **acromion process**, which is covered by the **middle fibres of the deltoid muscle**.
4. The **greater tubercle** forms the most lateral bony feature of the shoulder, being placed about 2 cm below the **lateral edge of the acromion process** beneath the **middle fibres of the deltoid** and lies in an anterior position and inferior to the **posterior angle of the acromion process**.
5. With the palpating fingertip on the **greater tubercle**, ask the model to rotate the **humerus**.
6. The **greater tubercle** of the **humerus** rotates under the palpating fingertip.

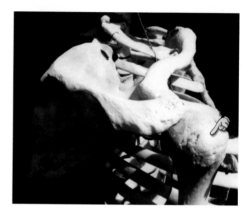

6. LESSER TUBERCLE OF HUMERUS

1. Identify the tip of the **coracoid process of the scapula** (*Objective No 3*).
2. Identify the **greater tubercle of the humerus** (*Objective No 5*).
3. Draw a horizontal line between the tip of the **coracoid process** and the **greater tubercle**.
4. Identify the **lesser tubercle of humerus** lying just below the midpoint of the horizontal line.
5. Palpate the **lesser tubercle of humerus** at this point in step 4 through the **anterior fibres of the deltoid**.
6. Ask the model to rotate the **humerus** with the palpating fingertip on the **lesser tubercle of humerus**.
7. The **lesser tubercle of humerus** can be identified as a rotating bony prominence through the **anterior fibres of the deltoid**.

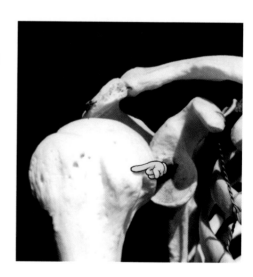

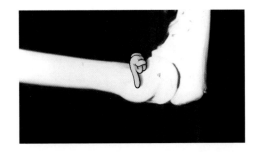

7. MEDIAL EPICONDYLE OF HUMERUS

1. Flex the **elbow joint** to a right angle.
2. Palpate with the tip of the index finger the midpoint of the medial surface of the **arm**.
3. Pass the tip of the index finger down the medial surface of the **arm** towards the **elbow** region.
4. The downwards movement of the palpating fingertip will come to rest at a prominent bony projection on the medial surface of the lower extremity of the **humerus**.
5. This prominent bony feature is the **medial epicondyle of humerus**.

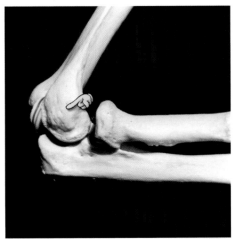

8. LATERAL EPICONDYLE OF HUMERUS

1. Flex the **elbow joint** to a right angle.
2. Apply firm pressure with the tip of the palpating index finger to the midpoint of the **arm** on the lateral surface.
3. At this midpoint on the lateral surface of the **arm** the mid shaft of the **humerus** can be palpated under the skin.
4. From this point palpate downwards on the lateral surface of the **arm** towards the **elbow** region.
5. On the lateral surface of the lower one-third of the **arm**, a bony ridge begins to become distinct under the palpating fingertip.
6. This distinct bony ridge is the **lateral supracondylar ridge of humerus**.
7. Continued palpation down this ridge leads directly to the lateral margin of the **lateral epicondyle of humerus** and its posterior surface.

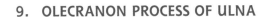

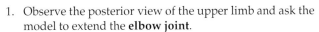

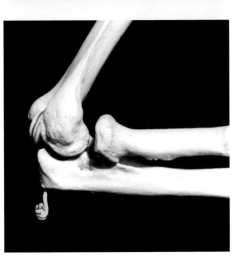

9. OLECRANON PROCESS OF ULNA

1. Observe the posterior view of the upper limb and ask the model to extend the **elbow joint**.
2. Surface mark with a pen on the posterior surface of the extended **elbow joint** the **lateral** and **medial epicondyles of the humerus** and join the two points with a horizontal line.
3. Palpate to the medial side of the midpoint of the horizontal line and a prominent bony process can be palpated under the skin.
4. This prominent bony process is the **olecranon process of ulna**.
5. Observe the posterior view of the **upper limb** and ask the model to flex the **elbow joint**.
6. Surface mark the position of the **medial and lateral epicondyles** as in step 2.
7. The **apex of olecranon process of ulna** descends when the **elbow joint** is flexed and forms an isosceles triangle with the **medial** and **lateral epicondyles of humerus**.

10.   HEAD OF ULNA

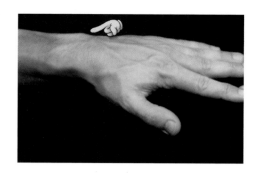

1. Ask the model to flex the **elbow joint** to a right angle and supinate the **forearm**.
2. Take the hand of the model and passively fully flex the **wrist joint**.
3. Fully flex the **elbow joint** and allow the fingertips of the passively flexed **wrist joint** to touch the **shoulder** and hold the position.
4. Observe the medial area of the **posterior aspect of the wrist**.
5. A prominent, elevated rounded projection of bone can be observed and palpated. Surface mark this anatomical feature, which is the **posterior aspect of the head of ulna**.
6. Immediately lateral to this projecting **head of ulna** is a depression. This depression is the **inferior radioulnar joint**.
7. Place a fingertip on the **head of ulna** and ask the model to supinate and pronate the **forearm**. Note the changing position of the **ulna** and **radius** forming the **inferior radioulnar joint**.
8. Place the hand back in the anatomical position and identify by palpation the rounded projection on the medial surface of the lower extremity of the **ulna** on the **posterior aspect of the wrist area** and surface mark with a pen.

11.   HEAD OF RADIUS

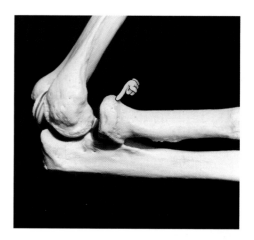

1. Observe the posterior view of the upper limb and ask the model to extend the **elbow joint**.
2. Identify and palpate a distinct depression on the lateral aspect of the midline.
3. Palpate the lateral aspect of the **olecranon process**, which is placed medially.
4. Palpate and surface mark the position of the posterior surface of the **lateral epicondyle**, which partly forms the depression in its upper area.
5. Palpate and surface mark the position of the posterior rounded surface of the **head of radius**, which partly forms the depression in its lower area.
6. Palpate and surface mark with a line the gap between the **head of radius** in the lower part of the depression and the **lateral epicondyle** in the upper part of the depression. This line represents the **humeroradial joint** line of the **elbow joint**.
7. Ask the model to flex the **elbow joint** to a right angle. Place a finger on the **head of radius** and note the movement of rotation when the model supinates and pronates the **radius**.

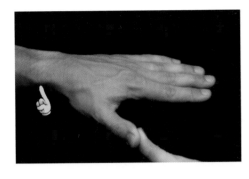

12. STYLOID PROCESS OF RADIUS

1. Ask the model to flex the **elbow joint** to a right angle.
2. Ask the model to place the **forearm** in a position midway between full pronation and supination with the **thumb** in full extension.
3. Observe the depression when the **thumb** is fully extended between the **tendons of the thumb extensors** on the **lateral aspect of the wrist** inferior to the raised projection made by the **lower extremity of the radius**.
4. Place a fingertip in this depression, known as the **anatomical snuffbox**, and palpate between the **extensor tendons of the thumb** moving proximally towards the expanded lower extremity of the **radius**.
5. The palpating fingertip will encounter a sharp pointed process of bone. This is the **styloid process of radius**.
6. Placing the palpating fingertip on the **styloid process of radius**, ask the model to move the **wrist joint** in radial and ulnar deviation.
7. The **styloid process of radius** may be identified as the proximal row of **carpal bones** move and the **styloid process** remains fixed.

13. STYLOID PROCESS OF ULNA

1. Identify by palpation and mark with a pen the prominent **head of ulna** (*Objective No 10*).
2. Mark a point inferior to the **head of ulna** on the posterior and medial surface.
3. The **styloid process** on the **head of ulna** lies at least 1 cm above a point corresponding to the **styloid process of radius**.

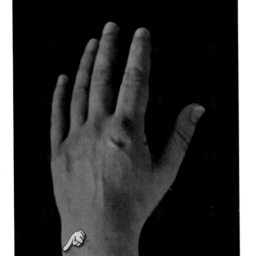

14. DORSAL TUBERCLE OF RADIUS

1. Ask the model to flex the **elbow joint** to a right angle and pronate the **forearm** to expose the **dorsum of the hand**.
2. Ask the model to fully extend the **thumb** and identify the tendon of **extensor pollicis longus**, tracing its course where it forms a boundary of the **anatomical snuffbox** to the **posterior surface of the radius**.
3. Maintain extension of the **thumb** and draw a line from the cleft between the **index** and **middle fingers** to the **posterior surface of the radius** to a point where the line forms a junction with the **tendon of extensor pollicis longus**.
4. Place a fingertip on this junction and a prominent tubercle can be distinguished.
5. The **tendon of extensor pollicis longus** passes round the medial aspect of this tubercle which is the **dorsal tubercle of the radius**.

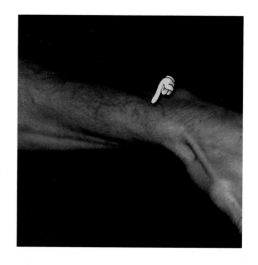

15. POSTERIOR BORDER OF SHAFT OF ULNA

1. Identify by palpation and mark the position of the **olecranon process of ulna**.
2. Draw a line from the prominent tip of the **olecranon process to the head of ulna**.
3. Identify by palpation a distinct subcutaneous ridge of bone along the course of the line marked from the tip of the **olecranon process** to the **head of ulna**.
4. This subcutaneous prominent ridge is the **posterior border of the shaft of ulna**.

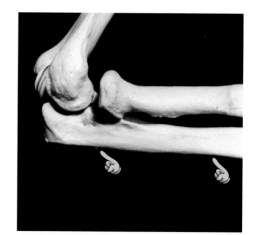

16. PISIFORM

1. Ask the model to flex the **elbow joint** to a right angle.
2. Identify by palpation the **head of ulna** (*Objective No 10*).
3. Move the fingertip round to the anteromedial surface of the **wrist** and ask the model to flex and ulnar deviate the **wrist joint** against maximal resistance.
4. Palpate the anteromedial surface of the **wrist** immediately proximal to the base of the **hypothenar eminence**.
5. Identify by palpation a distinct tendon at this point which appears to emanate at a small, round, pea-shaped bone. This is the **pisiform bone**.
6. Ask the model to pronate the **forearm** and passively flex the **wrist joint**.
7. Identify the **pisiform bone** and gently move it with a gliding action on the bone which lies posterior (**triquetral bone**).

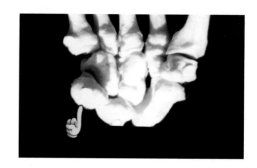

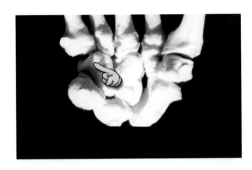

17. HAMATE

1. Ask the model to flex the **elbow joint** to a right angle.
2. Identify the **pisiform bone** (*Objective No 16*).
3. Palpate a point about 2.5 cm distal to the **pisiform bone** on the palmar surface of the hand in the direction of the cleft between the 4th and 5th fingers.
4. Apply firm pressure with the fingertip until a bony projection can be identified deep to the **hypothenar muscles**. This bony projection is the **hook of the hamate bone**.

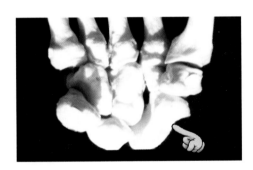

18. TRAPEZIUM

1. Ask the model to flex the **elbow joint** to a right angle.
2. Identify the position of the **scaphoid bone** (*Objective No 19*).
3. Place the tip of the palpating finger on the **scaphoid bone**.
4. Move the fingertip on the palmar surface of the **hand** about 2.5 cm in a fine line from the **scaphoid bone** to the cleft between **thumb** and **first finger**.
5. Palpate with firm pressure at this point deep to the **muscles of the thenar eminence**.
6. A crest-like projection of bone can be identified at this point.
7. This projection is the position of the **trapezium bone**.

19. SCAPHOID

1. Ask the model to flex the **elbow joint** to a right angle.
2. Ask the model to fully extend the **wrist joint**.
3. At the base of the **thenar eminence** directly distal to the **inferior extremity of the radius** the skin colour pales as a bone projects forwards during extension of the **wrist** against the skin.
4. This is the position of the **scaphoid bone**.
5. Identify the **styloid process of radius** (*Objective No 12*).
6. Palpate directly distal to the **styloid process of radius** in the **anatomical snuffbox**.
7. This is the position of the **scaphoid bone**.

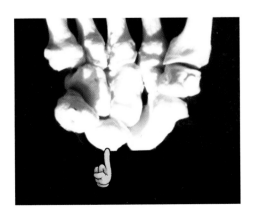

20. LUNATE

1. Ask the model to flex the **elbow joint** to a right angle.
2. Identify by palpation the **scaphoid bone**.
3. Identify by palpation and mark the **pisiform bone**.
4. Ask the model to flex the **wrist joint** against maximal resistance.
5. Identify the tendon of **palmaris longus**.
6. The tendon of **palmaris longus** crosses the **lunate bone**.
7. The **lunate bone** is positioned between the **pisiform** and **scaphoid bones**.

2

Joints of the Upper Limb

21. STERNOCLAVICULAR

1. Identify and mark the **jugular notch** on the superior border of the **manubrium**.
2. Move the fingertip about 4 mm in a lateral direction from the **jugular notch** until the prominent medial extremity of the **clavicle** is found.
3. Place the tip of the middle finger on the medial extremity of the **clavicle** and the tip of the index finger on the lateral edge of the **jugular notch**.
4. Ask the model to elevate and depress the shoulder; observe the movement taking place between the **sternum** and the **clavicle**.
5. Draw a line at the junction between the **manubrium** and the **clavicle** where movement is detected.

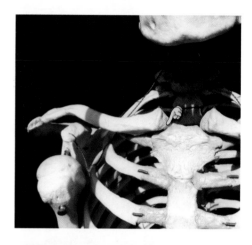

22. ACROMIOCLAVICULAR

1. Identify and mark the contour of the **acromion process of scapula**.
2. Place the index finger at a 45° angle on the **acromion process of scapula**, the tip of the index finger directed towards the **lateral extremity** of the **clavicle**.
3. Palpate in a medial direction until the prominent lateral extremity of the clavicle is found.
4. The **acromioclavicular joint** line lying in an anteroposterior direction is positioned under the tip of the index finger.
5. Distraction of the **glenohumeral joint** by manual traction along the long axis of the **shaft of humerus** produces passive movement at the **acromioclavicular joint**, which can be detected in a young adult.

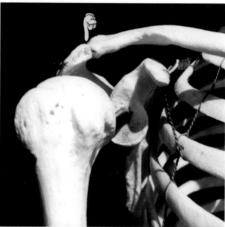

23. GLENOHUMERAL

1. Identify the tip of the **coracoid process**.
2. Draw a convex line downwards and outwards from a point just lateral to the tip of the **coracoid process** for 5 cm.
3. Draw a line with a slight concavity facing laterally to represent the lower edge of the **glenoid cavity** of the **shoulder joint**.

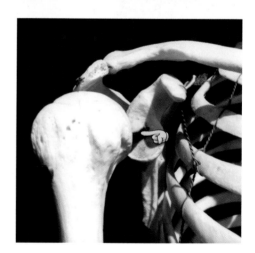

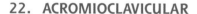

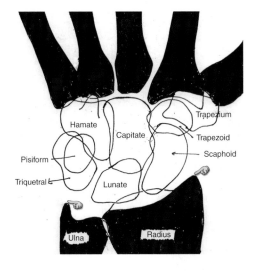

24. RADIOCARPAL

1. Identify and mark the tip of the **styloid process of radius**.
2. Identify and mark the **styloid process of ulna**.
3. Draw a line convex upwards from the tip of the **styloid process of radius** to the **styloid process of ulna** on the **anterior surface of the wrist**.
4. The lateral two-thirds of this line marks the line of the **radiocarpal joint**.

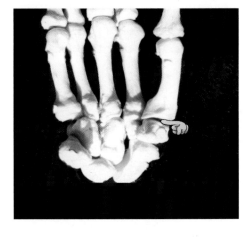

25. FIRST CARPOMETACARPAL

1. Identify and mark the **styloid process of radius**.
2. Identify and mark the anterior projection of the **scaphoid bone**.
3. Palpate and mark the lateral projection of the **scaphoid bone** in the **anatomical snuffbox** between the **tendons of extensor pollicis longus and brevis**.
4. Palpate and mark the lateral projection of the **trapezium bone** distal to the **scaphoid** in the **anatomical snuffbox**.
5. Palpate the prominent **base of the first metacarpal bone** immediately distal to the **trapezium** in the **anatomical snuffbox**.
6. Place the tip of the palpating finger on the **trapezium** and the **base of the first metacarpal bone**.
7. Ask the model to fully flex and extend the **thumb** while maintaining the position of the palpating fingertip in the **anatomical snuffbox**.
8. Detect the gliding movement at the joint between the **trapezium** and the **base of the first metacarpal bone of the thumb** and mark the joint line in the floor of the **anatomical snuffbox**.

26. SECOND METACARPOPHALANGEAL JOINT ON THE DORSAL SURFACE OF THE HAND

1. Ask the model to make a clenched fist with the right **hand**.
2. Mark the contour formed by the **head of the 2nd metacarpal bone**.
3. Ask the model to relax the **hand** so that the fingers may be passively moved.
4. Grasping the right **index finger** of the model, with the palmar surface of the examiner's fingers of the left hand in contact with the palmar surface of the right **index finger** of the model, apply gentle pain-free traction.
5. Gently flex the **finger joints** of the model's index finger to a right angle with the **palm**.
6. Ask the model to flex and extend the **index finger** while the examiner applies traction and resists the action of flexion and extension performed by the model.
7. The thumb tip of the examiner may be placed on the joint immediately distal to the **head of the 2nd metacarpal** where a gliding movement can be observed.
8. Mark on the dorsal surface of the **hand** where movement is taking place.
9. The line represents the dorsal surface marking of the **2nd metacarpophalangeal joint**.

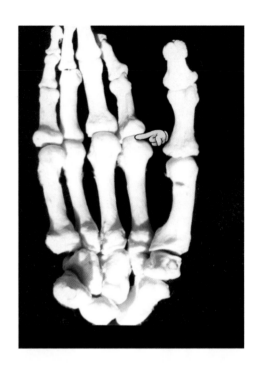

27. INTERPHALANGEAL

1. Ask the model to make a clenched fist with the right **hand**.
2. From the clenched fist position, ask the model to fully extend and flex the **index finger**.
3. Observe where the movement occurs between the **proximal**, **middle** and **distal phalanges of the index finger**.
4. Mark with a line on the dorsal surface of the **index finger** where this movement can be felt.
5. The lines on the dorsal surface of the **index finger** represent the position of the **interphalangeal joints**.

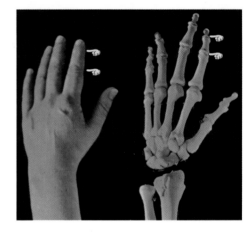

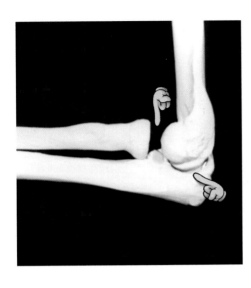

28. ELBOW

1. Identify and mark the **medial epicondyle of the humerus**.
2. Identify and mark the **lateral epicondyle of the humerus**.
3. Draw a horizontal line on the anterior surface of the **elbow** between the marked points steps 1 and 2.
4. Draw a horizontal line 2 cm inferior and parallel to the line in step 3.
5. This horizontal line shows the approximate surface marking of the **elbow joint**.
6. Ask the model to extend the **elbow joint** and palpate the **head of radius**.
7. Directly superior to the **head of radius** a depression can be palpated.
8. The horizontal line in step 5 should cut through this depression between the **head of radius** and the **capitulum of the humerus**, which forms the lateral component of the **elbow joint**.

3

Muscles of the Upper Limb

29. Trapezius
30. Latissimus dorsi
31. Rhomboids
32. Levator scapulae
33. Serratus anterior
34. Pectoralis major
35. Deltoid
36. Subscapularis
37. Supraspinatus
38. Infraspinatus
39. Teres minor
40. Teres major
41. Coracobrachialis
42. Biceps brachii
43. Brachialis
44. Triceps brachii
45. Pronator teres
46. Flexor carpi radialis
47. Flexor carpi ulnaris
48. Palmaris longus
49. Flexor digitorum superficialis
50. Flexor digitorum profundus
51. Flexor pollicis longus
52. Flexor retinaculum
53. Brachioradialis
54. Supinator
55. Extensor carpi radialis longus
56. Extensor carpi radialis brevis
57. Extensor digitorum
58. Extensor carpi ulnaris
59. Lateral intermuscular septum
60. Extensor digiti minimi
61. Extensor indicis
62. Abductor pollicis longus
63. Extensor pollicis brevis
64. Extensor pollicis longus
65. Abductor pollicis brevis
66. Adductor pollicis
67. Opponens pollicis
68. Flexor pollicis brevis
69. Abductor digiti minimi
70. Flexor digiti minimi
71. Opponens digiti minimi
72. Dorsal interossei
73. Palmar interossei

29. TRAPEZIUS

1. Palpate the bony lateral extremity of the **clavicle** and **acromion process of the scapula**.
2. Ask the model to maintain the anatomical position and to hold a 5 kg weight in one hand to demonstrate how the **upper fibres of trapezius** maintain the position of the distal extremity of the **clavicle and acromion process of the scapula** against the downward pull of the weight.
3. Palpate the medial one-third of the **spine of scapula**.
4. Ask the model to strongly adduct the **vertebral borders of the scapulae** towards the **median plane** to demonstrate the action of the **middle fibres of trapezius** working with the **rhomboid muscles**.
5. Ask the model to protract the **scapula** using **serratus anterior** and elevate the **upper limb** in the plane of the **scapula** against maximal resistance.
6. Palpate the **spine of scapula** and **fibres of trapezius** and note the movement and degrees of rotation of the **scapula** round the **thoracic wall** as the **upper limb** is placed in full elevation.
7. Palpate **trapezius** and note how the **upper**, **middle** and **lower fibres of trapezius** bring about **scapula** activity working with the **rhomboids** and **serratus anterior**.

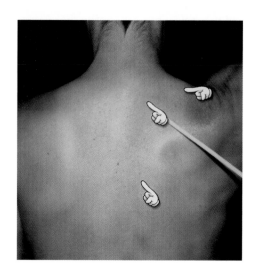

30. LATISSIMUS DORSI

1. Identify and surface mark the **inferior angle of scapula**.
2. Ask the model to sit down, place hands on knees and lean slightly forward.
3. Palpate the **inferior angle of scapula** and ask the model to cough.
4. Observe, palpate and surface mark the contraction and contour of **latissimus dorsi** as it passes over the **inferior angle of scapula** towards the posterior aspect of the axillary space and note how the muscle holds the **inferior angle of scapula** against the **thoracic wall** during coughing.
5. Ask the model to sit and grasp the seat of the chair with both hands, take both feet off the ground and, by strong extension of the **elbow joints**, lift the bodyweight from the chair seat.
6. Observe, palpate and surface mark the contraction of **latissimus dorsi** forming the posterior boundary of the axillary space as it extends and medially rotates the **glenohumeral joint**.
7. Ask the model to medially rotate, extend and adduct the **glenohumeral joint** and place a **hand** in a hip pocket to demonstrate the action of **latissimus dorsi**.
8. **Latissimus dorsi** is used by paraplegic patients when its nerve supply is intact.
9. **Latissimus dorsi** acts at a mechanical advantage when the **upper limb** is moving through a range of abduction of between 30 and 90°.
10. Note the action of this muscle in the down- and backstroke during swimming.

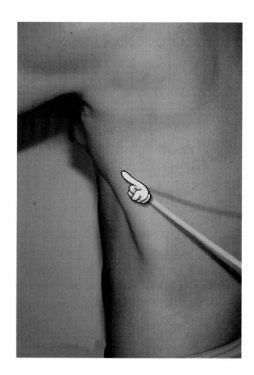

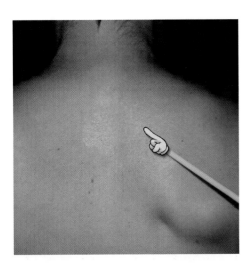

31. RHOMBOIDS

1. Palpate the bony prominence of the **vertebral border of scapula** between the **base of the spine of scapula** and the inferior angle.
2. Ask the model to strongly retract the vertebral borders of the **scapulae** towards the **median plane**.
3. Ask the model to abduct the **glenohumeral joint** and elevate the **scapula** against maximal resistance to demonstrate the action of **trapezius**.
4. The **rhomboid muscles** work as together with **trapezius** to rotate, elevate and adduct the **scapula** when the hand is raised above the head.
5. The **rhomboid muscles** cannot be palpated.

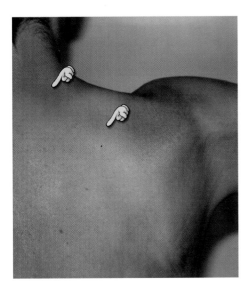

32. LEVATOR SCAPULAE

1. Ask the model to abduct the **glenohumeral joint** and elevate the **hand** above the **head**.
2. Palpate the bony vertebral border of the **scapula** between the **base of the spine of scapula** and **superior angle** as the model completes the activity and note the degree of elevation, rotation and slight protraction of the scapula.
3. The **levator scapulae muscle** cannot be palpated.

33. SERRATUS ANTERIOR

1. Ask the model to push strongly against resistance in the anatomical position. Ask the model to elevate the upper limb against resistance.
2. Palpate the **inferior angle of scapula** and note how it moves in rotation against the underlying **ribs**.
3. Palpate the **spine of scapula** and note how it moves forward in protraction and how the **scapula** is retained against the underlying ribs.
4. Observe and palpate the pronounced serrated digitations of **serratus anterior** on the **anterolateral aspect of the thoracic wall**.

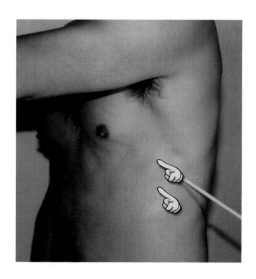

34. PECTORALIS MAJOR

1. Identify and surface mark the **clavicle**.
2. Identify and surface mark the **lateral margin of the sternum** and **costal cartilages 1–6**.
3. Ask the model to abduct the **glenohumeral joint** to 90°, place the **palms** together and strongly resist the movement of adduction towards the **median plane**.
4. Palpate immediately inferior to the medial two-thirds of the **shaft of clavicle** and identify the **clavicular attachment** of **pectoralis major**.
5. Palpate the **sternal attachment** of **pectoralis major** inferior to the **clavicular attachment** and lateral to the midline of the **sternum** and over the **costal cartilages 1–6**.
6. Palpate the anterior wall of the **axillary space**.
7. Resisted flexion of the **glenohumeral joint** accompanied by medial rotation and adduction accentuates the **clavicular attachment** of **pectoralis major**.
8. Resisted flexion with the **arm** in the horizontal plane accompanied by medial rotation and strong adduction accentuates the **sternal attachment** of **pectoralis major**.

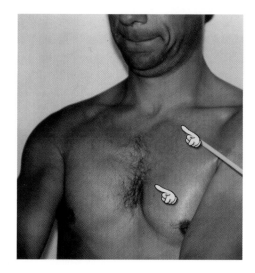

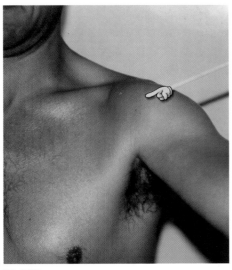

A

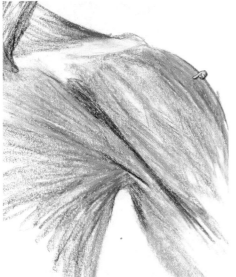

B

35. DELTOID

1. Identify and surface mark the lateral one-third of the **shaft of clavicle**, **acromion process** and the **spine of scapula**.
2. Ask the model to abduct the **glenohumeral joint** to 90°.
3. The **middle fibres of deltoid** can be palpated along the lateral margin of the **acromion process** passing towards the **deltoid tuberosity** on the lateral aspect of the **shaft of humerus**.
4. The **anterior fibres of deltoid** can be palpated inferior to the lateral one-third of the **shaft of clavicle** passing towards the **deltoid tuberosity** on the lateral aspect of the **shaft of humerus**.
5. The **posterior fibres of deltoid** can be palpated passing from the **spine of scapula** towards the **deltoid tuberosity** on the lateral aspect of the **shaft of humerus**.

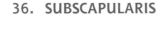

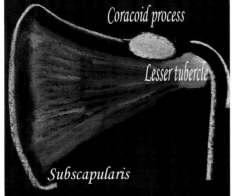

36. SUBSCAPULARIS

1. Ask the model to medially rotate and adduct the **glenohumeral joint**.
2. Ask the model to abduct the **arm** to 90° and medially rotate the **glenohumeral joint**.
3. The **tendon of subscapularis** passes high up in the **axillary space** to its attachment on the **lesser tubercle of humerus** and cannot be palpated.

37. SUPRASPINATUS

1. Palpate and surface mark the **spine of scapula, acromion process** and **greater tubercle of humerus**.
2. Ask the model to abduct the **glenohumeral joint** to 30° to demonstrate the action of **supraspinatus**.
3. Place the model in a sitting position with the **arm** fully supported in 90° of abduction to reduce muscle tone.
4. Gently palpate the **upper fibres of trapezius** immediately superior to the **spine of scapula** and move in a lateral direction towards the **greater tubercle of humerus** to identify the position of the **muscle** and **tendon of supraspinatus** proximal and then distal to the **acromion process** under which it has to pass to reach the **head of humerus**.

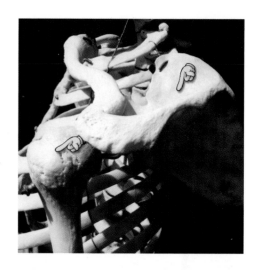

38 & 39. INFRASPINATUS AND TERES MINOR

1. Palpate and surface mark the **posterior fibres of deltoid**.
2. Palpate and surface mark the **axillary border of the scapula** immediately inferior to the **spine of scapula**.
3. Place the palm of one hand on the **scapula** to fix its position against the **thoracic wall**.
4. Ask the model to strongly laterally rotate and extend the **glenohumeral joint**.
5. Palpate the **posterior surface of the scapula** and **axillary border of the scapula**, moving in a lateral direction along a line directed towards a point medial to the **upper posterior fibres of deltoid**.

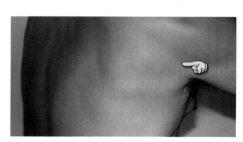

40. TERES MAJOR

1. Identify and surface mark the **inferior angle of scapula**.
2. Identify and surface mark the **superior border of latissimus dorsi** (*Objective No 30*) as it crosses the **inferior angle of scapula**.
3. Ask the model to adduct, extend and medially rotate the **glenohumeral joint**.
4. Palpate immediately superior and just lateral to the upper border of **latissimus dorsi** as it crosses the **inferior angle of scapula** in the area of **posterior wall** of the **axillary space**.

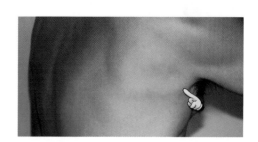

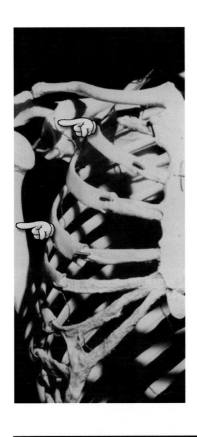

41. CORACOBRACHIALIS

1. Identify and surface mark the tip of the **coracoid process** (*Objective No 3*).
2. Identify and surface mark the position of the **deltoid tuberosity** on the lateral aspect of the **shaft of humerus**.
3. Mark a point opposite to the **deltoid tuberosity** on the medial aspect of the **shaft of humerus**.
4. Ask the model to adduct the **glenohumeral joint** with the **elbow joint** flexed as if holding a textbook in the **axillary space**.
5. Palpate the **contraction of coracobrachialis** from the tip of the **coracoid process** to the **anteromedial aspect** of the **upper one-third of the shaft of humerus** medial to the short head of **biceps brachii**.

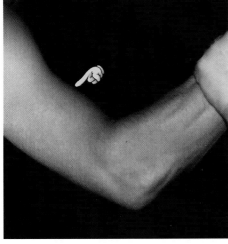

42. BICEPS BRACHII

1. Ask the model to flex the **elbow joint** to 90° and fully pronate the radioulnar joints so that the palm faces down.
2. Ask the model to grasp a small weight, supinate the **radioulnar joints**, flex the **elbow joint** and **glenohumeral joint**, following the sequence of bringing a spoon of food to the mouth.
3. The muscle belly of **biceps brachii** may be palpated on the **anteromedial surface of the humerus** approximately 8–10 cm above the line of the **elbow joint**.
4. The **distal tendon of attachment of biceps brachii** can be identified during the above movement as it passes over the **elbow joint** across the midline of the **cubital fossa** to the **bicipital tuberosity of radius**.
5. The pulse of the **brachial artery** can be identified medial to the **tendon of biceps brachii** in the **cubital fossa**.

43. BRACHIALIS

1. Ask the model to flex the **elbow joint** to 90° and fully pronate the **radioulnar joints** against maximal resistance.
2. **Brachialis** is positioned deep to **biceps brachii** and can be palpated lateral and posterior to the muscle belly of **biceps brachii** below the **deltoid tuberosity of humerus**.

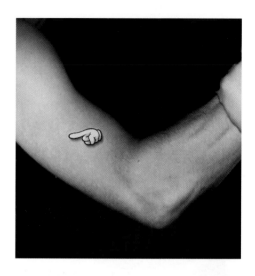

44. TRICEPS BRACHII

1. Identify and surface mark the **olecranon process of ulna** (*Objective No 9*).
2. Ask the model to fully flex the **elbow joint** and then extend against maximal resistance.
3. The three heads of **triceps brachii** occupy the posterior compartment of the **arm** and the muscle can be palpated on the posterior surface of the **arm** as it contracts during extension of the **elbow joint** and **glenohumeral joint**.
4. The **tendon of triceps brachii** forming the distal attachment can be palpated and traced to its insertion on the **olecranon process of ulna**.

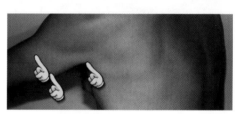

45. PRONATOR TERES

1. Ask the model to flex the **elbow joint** to 90° and fully supinate the **radioulnar joints**.
2. Ask the model to fully pronate the **radioulnar joints** against maximal resistance to place the **hand** with the palm facing down.
3. The **pronator teres** is a weak flexor of the **elbow joint** and works with **pronator quadratus**, a strong pronator, to bring about pronation.
4. **Pronator teres** may be palpated and is occasionally visible on the anterior surface of the **forearm** passing obliquely from the **medial epicondyle of humerus** and **coronoid process of ulna** towards the lateral surface of the **shaft of radius**.

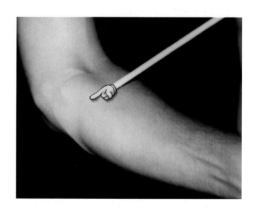

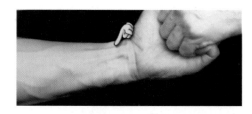

46. FLEXOR CARPI RADIALIS

1. Ask the model to flex the **elbow joint** to a right angle and supinate the **hand**.
2. Ask the model to flex and radially deviate the **radiocarpal joint** against maximal resistance applied to the palmar surface of the **hand**.
3. The subcutaneous **tendon of flexor carpi radialis** can be palpated and its position marked immediately lateral to the midline of the **forearm** on the anterior surface adjacent to the **tendon of palmaris longus**.

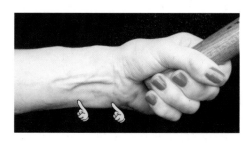

47. FLEXOR CARPI ULNARIS

1. Ask the model to flex the **elbow joint** to a right angle and supinate the **hand**.
2. Surface mark the position of the **pisiform bone** (*Objective No 16*).
3. Ask the model to flex and ulnar deviate the **radiocarpal joint** against maximal resistance applied to the palmar surface of the **hand**.
4. The subcutaneous **tendon of flexor carpi ulnaris** can be palpated and its position marked on the anteromedial surface of the **forearm** as it passes to its distal attachment on the **pisiform bone**.

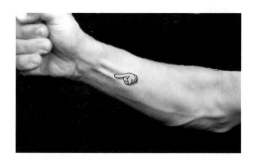

48. PALMARIS LONGUS

1. Ask the model to flex the **elbow joint** to a right angle and supinate the **hand**.
2. Ask the model to flex the **radiocarpal joint** and strongly oppose the tip of the **thumb** to the tip of the **5th finger**.
3. The long, distinct, subcutaneous **tendon of palmaris longus** crosses the anterior surface marking of the **radiocarpal joint** in the midline.
4. The **tendon of palmaris longus** lies medial to the **tendon of flexor carpi radialis**.
5. Research has shown that the **tendon of palmaris longus** is absent in 15% of the population.

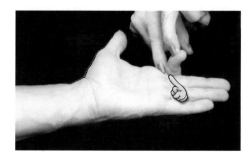

49. FLEXOR DIGITORUM SUPERFICIALIS

1. Ask the model to place a **hand** flat on a table with the palmar surface facing upwards.
2. Surface mark the **proximal phalanx** and the **proximal interphalangeal joint** of the index finger.
3. Ask the model to flex the **proximal interphalangeal joint** against maximal manual resistance.
4. During this movement the therapist isolates movement to the **proximal interphalangeal joint** by the application of manual resistance to the **proximal phalanx**.

50. FLEXOR DIGITORUM PROFUNDUS

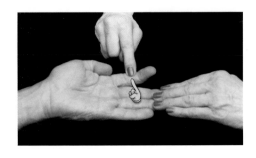

1. Ask the model to place a **hand** flat on a table with the palmar surface facing upwards.
2. Surface mark the **distal** and **middle phalanges** of the **index finger**.
3. Surface mark the **distal interphalangeal joint** of the **index finger**.
4. Ask the model to flex the **distal interphalangeal joint** against maximal manual resistance.
5. During this movement the therapist isolates movement to the **distal interphalangeal joint** by the application of manual resistance to the **middle phalanx**.

51. FLEXOR POLLICIS LONGUS

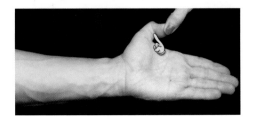

1. Ask the model to place the **hand** flat on a table with the palmar surface facing upwards.
2. Surface mark the **proximal phalanx**, **distal phalanx** and **interphalangeal joint** of the **thumb**.
3. Ask the model to flex the **interphalangeal joint** of the **thumb** against maximal manual resistance.
4. During this movement the therapist isolates movement to the **interphalangeal joint** of the **thumb** by the application of manual resistance to the **proximal phalanx** of the **thumb**.

52. FLEXOR RETINACULUM

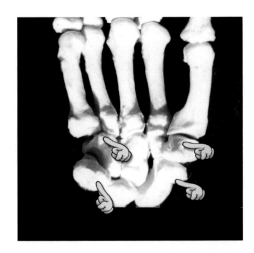

1. Ask the model to flex the **elbow joint** to a right angle and supinate the **hand**.
2. Surface mark the following carpal bones and anatomical features:
   a. **pisiform bone** and **hook of hamate**
   b. **tubercle of scaphoid** and **groove on trapezium**.
3. Draw a line connecting the **pisiform bone** and **hook of hamate** to represent the medial attachments.
4. Draw a line connecting the **tubercle of scaphoid** and **groove on trapezium** to represent the lateral attachments.
5. Complete the distal border surface marking of the **flexor retinaculum** by drawing a line to connect the **hook of hamate** and the **groove on trapezium**.
6. Complete the proximal border surface marking of the **flexor retinaculum** by drawing a line connecting the **pisiform bone** and the **tubercle of scaphoid**.
7. The area outlined should measure approximately 3 cm × 2.5 cm.

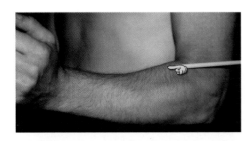

53. BRACHIORADIALIS

1. Ask the model to flex the **elbow joint** to 90°.
2. Ask the model to place the **hand** in the midway position between full pronation and full supination.
3. Apply maximal manual resistance to the lateral surface of the **forearm** proximal to the **styloid process of radius** (*Objective No 12*).
4. Ask the model to flex the **elbow joint** against resistance.
5. The prominent muscle belly of **brachioradialis** can be identified and palpated in the **upper two-thirds of the forearm** on the **anterolateral surface**.

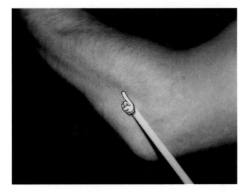

54. SUPINATOR

1. Ask the model to flex the **elbow joint** to 90° and fully pronate the **radioulnar joints**.
2. Identify and surface mark the position of the **head of radius** (*Objective No 11*).
3. Ask the model to fully supinate the **radioulnar joints** against maximal manual resistance.
4. Palpate the **head of radius** during supination and identify the position of the **neck of radius** which is placed immediately inferior to the **head of radius**.
5. The **supinator** passes round the **neck of radius** from its proximal attachments to the lateral surface of the upper one-third of the **shaft of radius** to which it inserts.

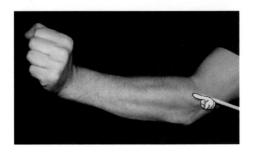

55. EXTENSOR CARPI RADIALIS LONGUS

1. Ask the model to flex the **elbow joint** to 90° and fully pronate the **forearm** with the palm facing down.
2. Fully extend the **radiocarpal joint** and produce a power grip against maximal resistance.
3. Maintain a few degrees of radial deviation.
4. Palpate and surface mark the **head, neck, shaft** and **base** of the **2nd metacarpal bone** of the **index finger**.
5. Palpate the dorsal surface of the **base of the 2nd metacarpal** and move a few millimetres in a proximal direction to a small depression immediately over the **distal row of carpal bones**.
6. Keeping in line with the **base of the 2nd metacarpal bone**, place the tip of the finger in this depression and ask the model to relax the power grip and then return to a power grip while maintaining the position of palpation.
7. The **tendon of extensor carpi radialis longus** can be palpated at this point as it passes to its distal attachment on the dorsal surface of the **base of the 2nd metacarpal bone** of the **index finger**.

56. EXTENSOR CARPI RADIALIS BREVIS

1. Ask the model to place a hand on a table with the dorsal surface facing upwards.
2. Surface mark the **head, neck, shaft** and **base of the 3rd metacarpal bone**.
3. Place the palpating fingertip on the dorsal surface of the **base of the 3rd metacarpal bone**.
4. Move the fingertip 3 mm in a proximal direction to palpate the **capitate bone**.
5. Maintaining the palpating fingertip on the **capitate bone**, ask the model to make a strong power grip with the radiocarpal joint held in extension and slight radial deviation.
6. The **tendon of extensor carpi radialis brevis** can be palpated as it passes to its distal attachment on the dorsal surface of the **base of the 3rd metacarpal bone**.
7. The **tendon of extensor carpi radialis brevis** lies medial to the **tendon of extensor carpi radialis longus** which passes to the dorsal surface of the **base of the 2nd metacarpal bone**.

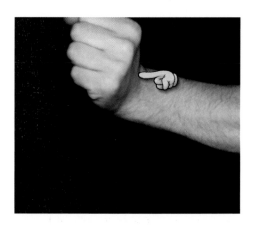

57. EXTENSOR DIGITORUM

1. Ask the model to place the **elbow, forearm** and **hand** on a table with the dorsal surface facing upwards and surface mark the **lateral epicondyle of humerus** (*Objective No 8*).
2. Ask the model to strongly extend the **radiocarpal, metacarpophalangeal** and **interphalangeal joints** of the **fingers** against maximal resistance.
3. The muscle belly can be clearly identified on the posterior surface of the **forearm** inferior to the **lateral epicondyle of humerus** adjacent to **extensor carpi radialis longus and brevis**.
4. The four **extensor tendons** of the **fingers** passing to their distal attachments on the **middle** and **distal phalanges** of each of the **four fingers** can be observed and palpated on the dorsal surface of the **hand** when the **proximal phalanges** are extended against maximal resistance.

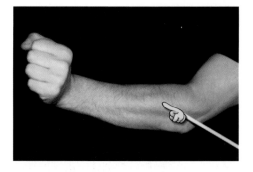

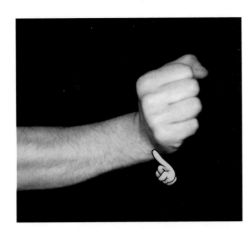

58. EXTENSOR CARPI ULNARIS

1. Ask the model to place a **hand** flat on a table with the palmar surface facing down.
2. Surface mark the **dorsal surface** of the **base of the 5th metacarpal bone**.
3. Surface mark the **lateral epicondyle of humerus** (*Objective No 8*) and **posterior border of ulna** (*Objective No 15*).
4. Ask the model to extend the **radiocarpal joint** and deviate towards the **ulna** against maximal resistance.
5. The muscle belly can be palpated inferior to the **lateral epicondyle of humerus**, on the posterior surface of the middle third of the **forearm**, lateral to the **posterior border of ulna**.
6. The **tendon of extensor carpi ulnaris** can be palpated passing to its distal attachment on the dorsal surface of the **base of the 5th metacarpal bone** immediately superior and then inferior to the **head of ulna** (*Objective No 10*).

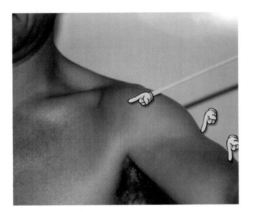

59. LATERAL INTERMUSCULAR SEPTUM

1. Surface mark the distal attachment of the **deltoid muscle** to the **deltoid tuberosity** on the lateral surface of the **shaft of humerus**.
2. Surface mark the **lateral epicondyle of humerus**.
3. Draw a vertical line connecting the **deltoid tuberosity** and the **lateral epicondyle of humerus**.
4. Mark a point to indicate the junction of the upper and middle thirds of the vertical line. (This is the point where the **radial nerve** passes through the **lateral intermuscular septum of the arm**.)
5. Draw an oblique line from the junction of the upper arm with the posterior boundary of the **axillary space**, through the point on the vertical line at step 4, and downwards and medially towards the lateral aspect of the **tendon of biceps brachii**.
6. The **radial nerve** can be palpated as it crosses the lateral aspect of the **midshaft of humerus** close to the surface.

60. EXTENSOR DIGITI MINIMI

1. Demonstrate and surface mark the muscle belly and main **tendon of extensor digitorum** prior to division into four separate tendons.
2. Demonstrate and surface mark the individual **tendon of extensor digitorum** passing to the **5th finger**.
3. Surface mark the **head of ulna**.
4. Ask the model to demonstrate **extensor digitorum** (*Objective No 57*) and palpate the individual **tendon** passing to the **5th finger** lateral to the **head of ulna**.
5. The **tendon of extensor digiti minimi** passing to unite with the **tendon of extensor digitorum** on its medial side can be identified at this point lateral to and inferior to the **head of ulna** and medial to the **tendon of extensor digitorum**.

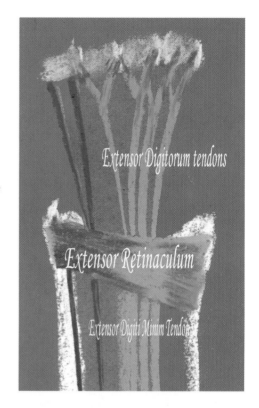

61. EXTENSOR INDICIS

1. Ask the model to make a loose fist, then extend the **radiocarpal joint**, and independently the **interphalangeal joints** of the **index finger** as in pointing the tip of the extended **finger** at an object.
2. The **extensor indicis** extends the **proximal phalanx** of the **index finger** and is an accessory extensor of the **radiocarpal joint**.
3. The **tendon of extensor indicis** joins with the individual **tendon** from the **extensor digitorum** to the **index finger** and reinforces the action of extending the **proximal phalanx of the index finger**.

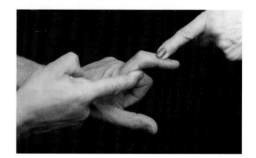

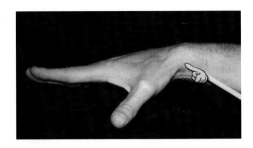

62. ABDUCTOR POLLICIS LONGUS

1. Ask the model to fully extend the **thumb joints** against maximal resistance with the **elbow joint** flexed to 90° and the **hand** in a position midway between the full range of pronation with the **thumb superior**.
2. Ask the model to maintain the position of the **thumb** in full extension, then to abduct the **thumb** to a position of full abduction, ensuring that the movement takes place in a direction that is at a right angle to the plane of the palm.
3. Observe the position of the **extensor pollicis brevis tendon** forming the anterior boundary of the **anatomical snuffbox**.
4. The **tendon of abductor pollicis longus** lies in a position which is parallel and immediately anterior to the **tendon of extensor pollicis brevis** as it passes to its distal attachment on the lateral surface of the **base of the 1st metacarpal bone of the thumb**.

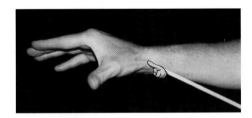

63. EXTENSOR POLLICIS BREVIS

1. Ask the model to fully extend the **1st phalanx of the thumb** against maximal resistance, with the **elbow joint** flexed to 90° and the **hand** in a position midway between the full range of pronation with the **thumb superior**.
2. The **tendon of extensor pollicis brevis** forms the anterior boundary of the **anatomical snuffbox** which can be clearly demonstrated when the **extensor pollicis longus** and **extensor pollicis brevis** work together to fully extend the **joints of the thumb**.
3. Palpate the **tendon of extensor pollicis brevis** where it forms the anterior boundary of the **anatomical snuffbox** as it passes to its distal attachment on the dorsal surface of the base of the **first phalanx of the thumb**.

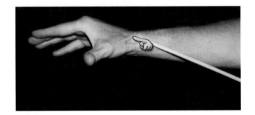

64. EXTENSOR POLLICIS LONGUS

1. Ask the model to fully extend the **thumb joints** against maximal resistance with the **elbow joint** flexed to 90° and the **hand** placed in a position midway between the full range of pronation with the **thumb superior**.
2. The distinct subcutaneous **long tendon of extensor pollicis longus** forms the posterior boundary of the **anatomical snuffbox** which is clearly visible when the **thumb joints** are fully extended.
3. The **long tendon** can be palpated from where it passes round the **dorsal tubercle of radius** (*Objective No 14*) to its distal attachment on the dorsal surface of the base of the **distal phalanx of the thumb**.

65. ABDUCTOR POLLICIS BREVIS

1. Ask the model to place a **hand** on a table with the palmar surface facing upwards.
2. Surface mark the position of the base of the **proximal phalanx of the thumb**.
3. Surface mark the position of the **trapezium** (*Objective No 18*).
4. Ask the model to abduct the **thumb** at a right angle to the **plane of the palm** against maximal resistance.
5. The belly of **abductor pollicis brevis** can be palpated on the **anterolateral aspect of the thenar eminence** as its fibres pass to the lateral aspect of the base of the **proximal phalanx of the thumb**.

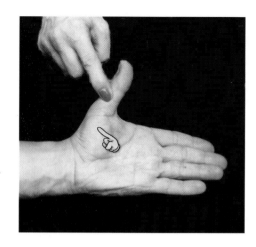

66. ADDUCTOR POLLICIS

1. Ask the model to place a **hand** on a table with the palmar surface facing upwards.
2. Ask the model to abduct the **thumb** at a right angle to the plane of the palm and hold the position.
3. Ask the model to adduct the **thumb** at a right angle to the plane of the palm against maximal resistance in a direction towards the **index finger**.
4. The muscle belly can be palpated on the **anteromedial** surface of the **metacarpophalangeal joint** of the **thumb** as it passes towards its distal attachment on the medial aspect of the base of the **proximal phalanx of the thumb**.

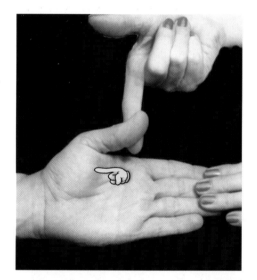

67. OPPONENS POLLICIS

1. Ask the model to place a **hand** on a table with the palmar surface facing upwards.
2. Surface mark the position of the **trapezium**.
3. Surface mark the shaft of the **1st metacarpal bone**.
4. Ask the model to bring together the tip of the **thumb** to the tip of the **little finger** in the action of opposition using maximal resistance.
5. The **opponens pollicis brevis** lies medial to **flexor pollicis brevis** in the **thenar eminence**.
6. The muscle belly can be palpated along the anterior surface of the shaft of the **1st metacarpal bone** as it passes to its distal attachment.

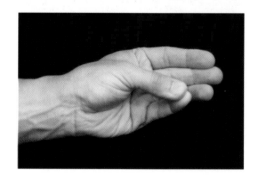

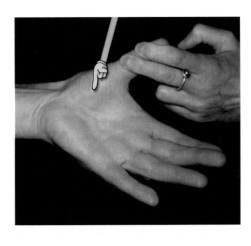

68. FLEXOR POLLICIS BREVIS

1. Ask the model to place a **hand** on a table with the palmar surface facing upwards.
2. Surface mark the position of the **trapezium** (*Objective No 18*) and the shaft of the **1st metacarpal bone**.
3. Surface mark the position of the **base of the proximal phalanx of the thumb**.
4. Ask the model to flex the **proximal phalanx of the thumb** parallel to the plane of the palm against maximal resistance.
5. Part of the muscle belly of **flexor pollicis brevis** may be palpated on the medial aspect of **abductor pollicis brevis** as it passes to its distal attachments on each side of the base of the **proximal phalanx of the thumb**.

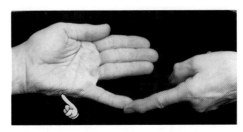

69. ABDUCTOR DIGITI MINIMI

1. Ask the model to place a **hand** on a table with the palmar surface facing upwards.
2. Surface mark the **pisiform bone** and base of the **proximal phalanx of the little finger**.
3. Ask the model to abduct the **little finger** against maximal resistance maintaining the **middle and distal phalanges** in extension.
4. The muscle belly of **abductor digiti minimi** may be palpated on the medial border of the **hypothenar eminence** from the **pisiform bone** to its distal attachment on the **medial aspect of the base of the proximal phalanx** of the **little finger**.

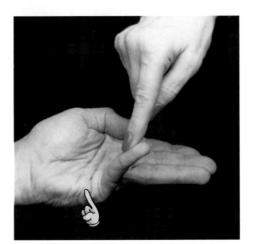

70. FLEXOR DIGITI MINIMI

1. Ask the model to place a **hand** flat on a table with the palmar surface facing upwards.
2. Surface mark the position of the **hook of the hamate bone** (*Objective No 17*) and the medial aspect of the base of the **proximal phalanx of the little finger**.
3. Ask the model to flex the **metacarpophalangeal joint of the little finger** against maximal resistance with the **interphalangeal joints** maintained in extension.
4. The muscle belly of **flexor digiti minimi** may be palpated lateral and adjacent to the muscle belly of **abductor digiti minimi** as it passes from the **hook of the hamate bone** to its distal attachment on the medial aspect of the **base of the proximal phalanx of the little finger**.

71. OPPONENS DIGITI MINIMI

1. Ask the model to place a **hand** on a table with the palmar surface facing upwards.
2. Surface mark the position of the **hook of the hamate bone** (*Objective No 17*).
3. Surface mark the position of the medial border of the shaft of the **5th metacarpal bone**.
4. Ask the model to bring the tip of the **little finger** and tip of the **thumb** together using firm pressure in the action of opposition.
5. The belly of **opponens digiti minimi** lies lateral to **flexor digiti minimi** and can be palpated with deep pressure on the **hypothenar eminence** as it passes from the **hook of hamate** to its distal attachment on the medial border of the **5th metacarpal bone**.

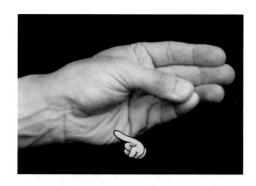

72. DORSAL INTEROSSEI

1. Ask the model to extend the **radiocarpal joint**, flex the **metacarpophalangeal joint**, and extend the **interphalangeal joints of the fingers**.
2. Ask the model to maintain this position and abduct the **index finger** from the midline of the **hand** towards the **thumb**.
3. The belly of the **1st dorsal interosseous muscle** can be palpated in the interval between the **1st and 2nd metacarpal bones** as the **index finger** is abducted from the midline.

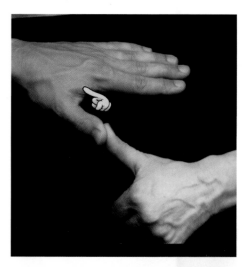

73. PALMAR INTEROSSEI

1. Ask the model to extend the **radiocarpal joint**, flex the **metacarpophalangeal joint** and extend the **interphalangeal joints of the fingers**.
2. Place a sheet of paper between the extended **fingers** and ask the model to hold the paper in position.
3. Maintaining the position, ask the model to adduct the **fingers** towards the midline and resist the removal of the sheet of paper held between the adducted **fingers**.
4. The action of both sets of **interossei** is demonstrated in the daily activity of writing a letter when they work with the **lumbrical muscles** to bring about the required movements at the **metacarpophalangeal** and **interphalangeal joints**.

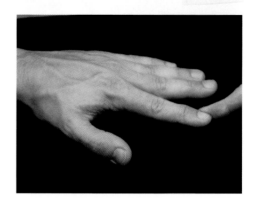

Superficial Veins of the Upper Limb

74. CEPHALIC

1. Note the dorsal venous network on the dorsum of the **hand**.
2. Mark the **cephalic vein** where it drains the dorsal surface of the **hand** on the lateral aspect at the base of the **thumb** and winds round the **wrist** to gain the anterior surface of the **forearm**.
3. The **cephalic vein** ascends on the radial side of the **forearm** to gain the **cubital fossa**.
4. The **cephalic vein** lies in the sulcus on the lateral aspect of **biceps brachii** and ascends the **arm**.
5. The **cephalic vein** passes between the **deltoid muscle** and the **pectoralis major** (*Objectives Nos 34 and 35*) to pierce fascia immediately inferior to the **shaft of clavicle**.
6. Ask the model to flex and adduct the **shoulder joint** against resistance to demonstrate the action of the **anterior fibres of deltoid** and **pectoralis major**.
7. The **cephalic vein** passes through this triangle to pierce fascia and joins the **axillary vein**.
8. Mark this triangular space named the **delto-pectoral triangle**.

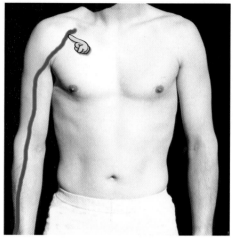

A

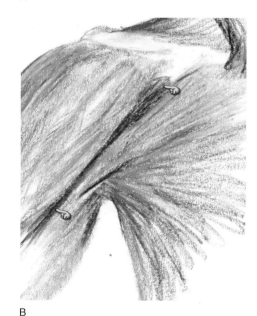

B

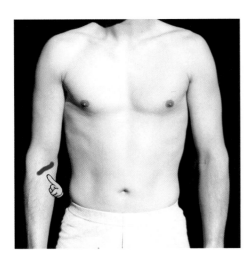

75. MEDIAN CUBITAL

1. Identify and mark the **cephalic vein** (*Objective No 74*) in the roof of the **cubital fossa**.
2. Identify and mark the **basilic vein** (*Objective No 76*) in the roof of the **cubital fossa**.
3. Draw a line ascending from the **cephalic vein** crossing the **cubital fossa** to join the **basilic vein**.
4. This line communicating with the **cephalic** and **basilic veins** in the roof of the **cubital fossa** represents the **median cubital vein**.
5. The **cephalic**, **basilic** and **medial cubital veins** form the letter M in the **cubital fossa**.
6. When the superficial venous blood flow is restricted by light pressure to the **upper limb**, these veins are made prominent.

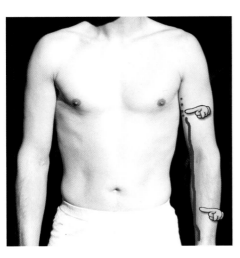

76. BASILIC

1. Note the **dorsal venous network** on the dorsum of the **hand**.
2. Mark the **basilic vein** on the dorsum of the **hand** on the medial aspect close to the base of the **2nd metacarpal bone**.
3. The **basilic vein** winds round the medial side of the **wrist** to gain the anterior surface of the **forearm**.
4. The **basilic vein** ascends the **forearm** on the ulnar side to gain the **cubital fossa**.
5. The **cephalic vein** ascends lying in a sulcus on the medial side of the **biceps brachii muscle**.
6. At a point midway between the **medial epicondyle of humerus** and the tip of the **coracoid process of scapula** on the medial side of the **arm**, the **basilic vein** pierces fascia and becomes the **axillary vein**.

5

Arterial Pulses of the Upper Limb

77. AXILLARY ARTERY

1. Ask the model to abduct the **arm** through 90° and laterally rotate the **shoulder joint**.
2. Identify the lateral border of the body of the **1st rib** in the **supraclavicular fossa** (*Objective No 164*).
3. Draw a line from the midpoint of the **shaft of clavicle** and the lateral border of the **1st rib** which lies immediately posterior.
4. Complete the line from step 3 to a point representing the junction of the anterior and middle thirds of the lateral wall of the **axillary space**.
5. This line passes medial to the tip of the **coracoid process of scapula**.
6. Count the pulse of the **axillary artery** immediately medial to the tip of the **coracoid process**.

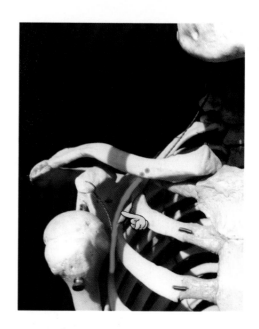

78. BRACHIAL ARTERY

1. Ask the model to abduct the arm through 90° and laterally rotate the **shoulder joint**.
2. Palpate and surface mark the **head of radius** (*Objective No 11*).
3. Palpate the lateral boundary of the **axillary space** (*Objective No 206*).
4. Mark the position of the **axillary artery** at a point representing the junction of the anterior and middle thirds of the **lateral boundary** of the **axillary space**.
5. At this point the artery name is changed from **axillary** to **brachial**.
6. Count the pulse of the **axillary artery** at this point where it can be compressed against the underlying medial surface of the shaft of **humerus**.
7. Identify the **cubital fossa** and surface mark the anterior line of the **elbow joint** (*Objective No 28*).
8   Mark the midpoint of the line at the level of the **head of radius**.
9. Draw a line from the marked points in step 4 to step 8.
10. Note the projected line lies on the medial surface of **biceps brachii** and the tendon of **biceps brachii** at the **elbow joint**.
11. Count the pulse of the **brachial artery**.

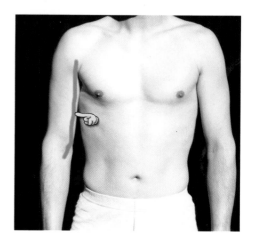

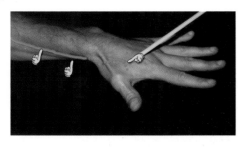

79. RADIAL ARTERY

1. Identify the **head of radius** and surface mark the projected position on the anterior surface of the **forearm**.
2. Mark a point on the anterior surface of the lower quarter of the **forearm** immediately lateral to the **tendon of flexor carpi radialis** proximal to the base of the **thenar eminence** (*Objective No 46*).
3. Connect the marked points in steps 1 and 2 with a line.
4. Count the pulse of the **radial artery**.

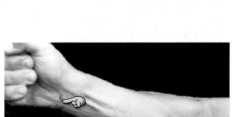

80. ULNAR ARTERY

1. Identify the anterior surface marking of the **elbow joint** and mark (*Objective No 28*).
2. Identify the midpoint and mark at the level of the **head of radius** (*Objective No 11*).
3. Identify the **pisiform bone** (*Objective No 16*) and mark a point immediately proximal and lateral on the anterior surface adjacent to the **pisiform bone**.
4. Draw a line from the marked points in step 2 to step 3.
5. Count the pulse of the **ulnar artery** lying lateral to the **pisiform bone** and the tendon of **flexor carpi ulnaris** (*Objective No 47*).

Peripheral Nerves of the Upper Limb

81. MEDIAN NERVE AT THE ELBOW OR WRIST

1. Identify the pulse of the **brachial artery** on the medial aspect of the **biceps brachii** in the medial compartment of the **cubital fossa** (*Objective No 203*).
2. Mark the position of the pulse of the **brachial artery** in the **cubital fossa**.
3. Place a mark immediately medial to the **biceps brachii tendon** at the level of the base of the **cubital fossa** to indicate the position of the **median nerve**.
4. Identify the **tendon of palmaris longus** as it crosses the anterior surface marking of the **radiocarpal joint** (*Objective No 48*).
5. Place a mark immediately lateral to the tendon of **palmaris longus** at the level of the **radiocarpal joint**.
6. Identify the **tendon of flexor carpi radialis** at the level of the **radiocarpal joint** and surface mark (*Objective No 46*).
7. The **median nerve** lies immediately lateral to the **tendon of palmaris longus** as it crosses the anterior surface marking of the **radiocarpal joint** and 1 cm medial to the **tendon of flexor carpi radialis**. Surface mark this point.
8. A line drawn on the surface joining points marked in steps 3 and 7 indicates the projected course of the **median nerve** at the level of the **elbow joint** to the **radiocarpal joint**.

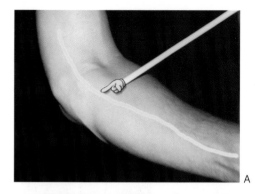

A

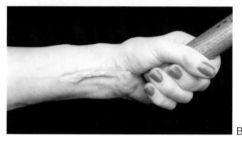

B

82. AXILLARY/CIRCUMFLEX NERVE

1. Draw a vertical line from the midpoint of the lateral border of the **acromion process** (*Objective No 4*) to the distal attachment (**deltoid tubercle/tuberosity**) of the **deltoid muscle** on the lateral aspect of the **shaft of humerus**.
2. Draw a horizontal line at right angles to the long axis of the **humerus** at a point midway on the vertical line in step 1.
3. This horizontal line represents the course of the **axillary/circumflex nerve** as it crosses the **surgical neck of humerus**.

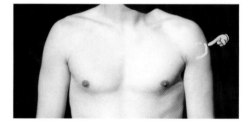

83. ULNAR NERVE AT THE ELBOW OR WRIST

1. Identify and mark the **medial epicondyle of humerus** and **olecranon process of ulna** (*Objectives Nos 7 and 9*).
2. Mark a point in the **sulcus** between the **medial epicondyle of humerus** and **olecranon process of ulna**.
3. Identify and mark the position of the **pisiform bone** (*Objective No 16*).
4. Identify and mark the position of the **tendon of flexor carpi ulnaris** at the level of the **wrist joint** (*Objective No 47*).
5. Identify and mark the position of the **ulnar artery pulse** lateral to the **tendon of flexor carpi ulnaris**.
6. Mark a point lateral to the **pisiform bone** and **tendon of flexor carpi ulnaris** but medial to the position of the **ulnar artery** at the level of the **wrist joint**.
7. Join points marked in steps 2 and 6 with a line.
8. This line represents the projected course of the **ulnar nerve** from the **elbow joint** to the **wrist joint**.

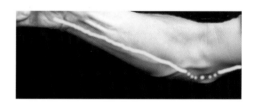

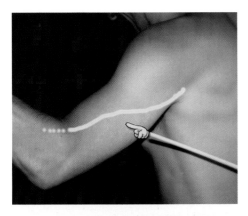

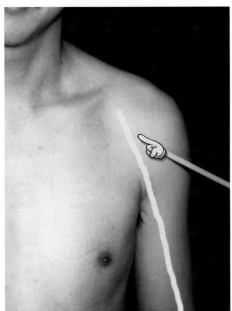

84. RADIAL NERVE IN THE ARM OR AT THE ELBOW

1. Draw a vertical line on the lateral surface of the **arm** from the distal attachment of the **deltoid muscle** (*Objective No 35*) to the **lateral epicondyle of humerus** (*Objective No 8*).
2. Mark a point on the line at the junction of the upper and middle thirds.
3. Draw a line from the posterior boundary of the **axillary space**, downwards and laterally to the point in step 2.
4. Continue the line from the point in step 2, downwards on the lateral aspect of the tendon of **biceps brachii** to the **lateral epicondyle** towards the **head of radius** and stop at the **neck of radius**.

85. MUSCULOCUTANEOUS NERVE IN THE ARM

1. Identify and mark the tip of the **coracoid process of scapula**. (*Objective No 3*).
2. Mark a point 3 cm inferior to the tip of the **coracoid process**.
3. Draw a line from the marked point in step 2 to the lateral **bicipital sulcus** immediately superior to the **lateral epicondyle of humerus**.
4. The line cuts across the contours of **coracobrachialis**, **biceps brachii** and **brachialis** and represents the projected course of the **musculocutaneous nerve** in the **arm**.

7

Bony Features of the Lower Limb

86. Iliac crest
87. Greater trochanter of femur
88. Ischial tuberosity
89. Sacrum
90. Medial condyle of femur
91. Adductor tubercle of femur
92. Medial condyle of tibia
93. Lateral outline of lateral condyle of femur
94. Lateral condyle of tibia
95. Borders of the patella
96. Head of fibula
97. Neck of fibula
98. Tibial tuberosity

99. Medial process of calcaneal tuberosity
100. Anterior border of the shaft of tibia
101. Medial malleolus
102. Peroneal tubercle
103. Lateral malleolus
104. Tuberosity of navicular
105. Sustentaculum tali
106. Head and neck of talus
107. Cuboid bone
108. Medial cuneiform bone
109. Bone of the 5th metatarsal bone of the foot

86. ILIAC CREST

1. Ask the model to lie down in the **supine position.** Place the **hands** one on each side of the midline below the transpyloric plane with the palmar surfaces on the antero-lateral abdominal wall, finger tips facing in a lateral direction. The tip of the little finger will rest on or close to the bony prominence of the **anterior superior iliac spine.**

2. The **anterior superior iliac spine** marks the anterior commencement of the **iliac crest** and in a model is clearly visible below the skin.

3. Palpate the **anterior superior iliac spine** and move upwards and in a posterior direction along the **iliac crest** for about 5 cm until a prominent bony feature can be palpated between the fingertip and the thumb. This feature is the **tubercle of the crest.**

4. A line drawn between the **tubercles of the iliac crest** cuts the upper border of the spinous process of the **5th lumbar vertebra.**

5. Continue palpating along the **iliac crest**. The midpoint between the **anterior superior iliac spine** and the termination of the **iliac crest** at the **posterior superior iliac spine** is reached.

6. The palpating fingertip continues to rise as it moves along the **iliac crest** and the summit is reached.

7. A line drawn between the summits of the **iliac crests** cuts through an interval between the **spinous processes of the 3rd and 4th lumbar vertebrae.**

8. Continue palpating as the **iliac crest** descends and to trace it medially to its termination at the **posterior superior iliac crest.**

9. A dimple, 5 cm from the median plane, which overlies the **posterior superior iliac spine**, indicates the position of the **posterior superior iliac spine.**

10. A line drawn between the two dimples marking the position of the **posterior superior iliac spines** cuts through the body of the **2nd sacral vertebra.**

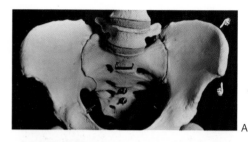

A

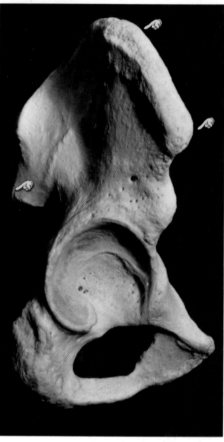

B

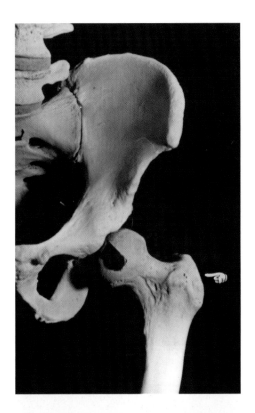

87. GREATER TROCHANTER OF FEMUR

1. Identify and surface mark the **anterior superior iliac spine** of the **iliac crest**.
2. Identify and surface mark the most prominent point of the **ischial tuberosity**.
3. Draw a line from the **anterior superior iliac spine** to the most prominent point of the **ischial tuberosity**.
4. The line drawn crosses the superior aspect of the greater **trochanter of femur** and the centre of the **acetabulum** of the **innominate bone** forming the **hip joint**.
5. The **greater trochanter of femur** is subcutaneous in its inferior part and presents a quadrilateral bony shape.
6. Place the palm of the model on the lateral aspect of the **hip** area with the fingertips parallel and together facing in an anterior direction and the thumb resting just **inferior to the iliac crest**.
7. The medial border of the 5th finger is placed superior to the **subcutaneous quadrilateral prominent bony mass** of the **greater trochanter of femur**.

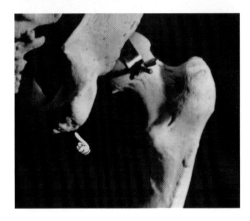

88. ISCHIAL TUBEROSITY

1. Ask the model to slowly flex the **hip joints** and assume a sitting position on their palms with the **fingertips** facing towards the median plane.
2. As the thighs of the model reach the horizontal position, the palmar surfaces of the **fingertips** are able to palpate a prominent bony mass which becomes subcutaneous as the **lower fibres of gluteus maximus** pass in a lateral direction.
3. The prominent bony feature exposed to palpation is the **ischial tuberosity**.
4. On extending the **hip joints** and rising back to regain the anatomical position, the **ischial tuberosity** is covered by the **lower fibres of gluteus maximus**.

89. SACRUM

1. Identify and surface mark the **posterior superior iliac spines**.
2. Observe that the **posterior superior iliac spines** lie 5 cm from the **median plane**.
3. Draw a line between the two **posterior superior iliac spines**.
4. Note that the line cuts through the body of the **2nd sacral spinous process**.
5. Observe the **natal cleft** and the inverted triangle formed between the two dimples overlying the **posterior superior iliac spines** and the **natal cleft**.
6. The tip of the **apex of the natal cleft** lies on a level with the **3rd sacral spine**.
7. Join the points marking the dimples to form the base of a triangle and the tip of the **natal cleft** to form the apex.
8. The **sacral hiatus** can be located inferior of the triangle apex.
9. The **1st sacral vertebra** is located superior to the horizontal line joining the dimples overlying the **posterior superior iliac spines**.
10. Note that the **posterior superior iliac spine** lies over the midpoint of a line indicating the surface marking of the **sacroiliac joint**.

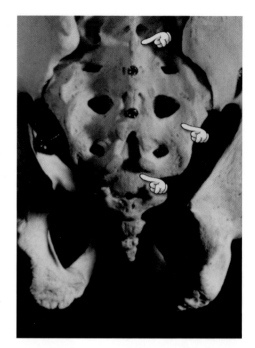

90. MEDIAL CONDYLE OF FEMUR

1. Ask the model to sit down.
2. Flex the **knee joint** passively to a right angle.
3. Place the palpating fingertips on the medial aspect of the **thigh** and with firm pressure palpate downwards towards the **knee joint**.
4. The **medial condyle of femur** presents as a large mass of bone which flares out from the **medial surface** of the lower extremity of the **shaft of femur**.
5. The medial and slightly projecting anterior surface can be identified lying medial to **medial border of the patella**.
6. The **anteromedial compartment** and line of the **knee joint** can be palpated as a subcutaneous space between the **medial condyles of femur and tibia**.
7. The posterior surface of the **medial condyle of femur** is obscured by muscle tendons and joint structures.

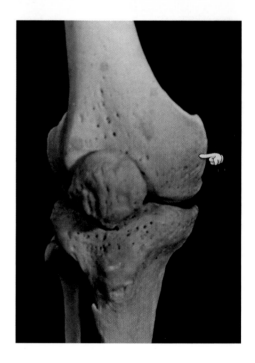

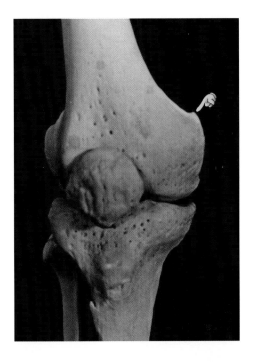

91. ADDUCTOR TUBERCLE OF FEMUR

1. Identify the highest point on the **medial condyle of femur** (*Objective No 90*).
2. Place the palmar surfaces of the palpating fingers on the **medial aspect of the thigh**.
3. Palpate with firm pressure in a downwards direction towards the highest point of the **medial condyle of femur**.
4. The tip of the middle finger will come into contact with the **adductor tubercle of the femur**.
5. Ask the model to adduct the **hip joint** with resistance applied to the **adductor tubercle**.
6. The strong cord-like **tendon of adductor magnus** can be identified passing downwards to its **distal attachment on the femur**.

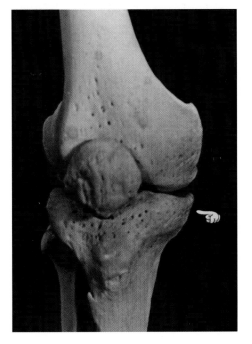

92. MEDIAL CONDYLE OF TIBIA

1. Ask the model to sit down.
2. Identify and mark the outline of the **patella** (*Objective No 95*).
3. Place the tip of the index finger on the **medial border of the patella** and move medially to identify the **anteromedial depression** indicating the underlying anterior compartment of the **knee joint**.
4. The subcutaneous bony edge of the **tibial plateau** can be identified forming the inferior border of the depression and the upper limit of the **medial condyle of tibia**.
5. Below this bony edge the prominent mass of the **medial condyle of tibia** can be palpated.

93. LATERAL OUTLINE OF LATERAL CONDYLE OF FEMUR

1. Ask the model to sit down.
2. Identify and mark the **contour of the head of fibula** (*Objective No 96*).
3. Palpate with the fingertip the subcutaneous bony edge of the **tibial plateau** lying approximately 1 cm superior and slightly anterior to the **head of fibula**.
4. The subcutaneous bony edge of the **tibial plateau** forms the inferior boundary of the **anterolateral** compartment of the **knee joint** which can be palpated immediately lateral to the lateral border of the **patella**.
5. Immediately above the **anterolateral compartment** of the **knee joint** lies the prominent bony mass of the **lateral condyle of femur**.

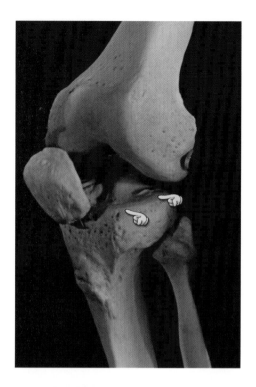

94. LATERAL CONDYLE OF TIBIA

1. Ask the model to sit down.
2. Identify the **head of fibula** (*Objective No 96*).
3. Palpate the bony subcutaneous edge of the **tibial plateau** approximately 1 cm superior and slightly anterior to the **head of fibula**.
4. Trace the **edge of the tibial plateau** to the lateral border of the **ligamentum patellae**.
5. Below this edge, overhanging the **shaft of tibia**, lies the mass of the prominent **lateral condyle of tibia**.

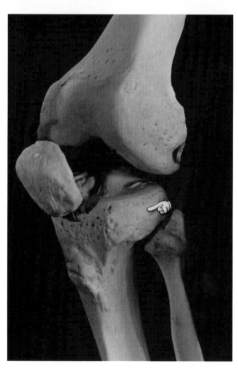

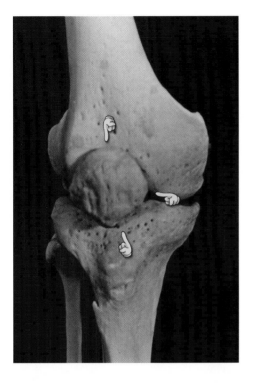

95. BORDERS OF THE PATELLA

1. Ask the model to lean forwards slightly from standing to reduce the muscle tone in **quadriceps femoris**.
2. Grasp the **patella** between the tip of the index finger and the thumb. Move the **patella** passively over the anterior surfaces of the **femoral condyles**.
3. Note that the inferior pole of the **patella** lies 1 cm above the line of the **knee joint**.
4. Palpate the inferior pole of the **patella** and trace the **ligamentum patellae** down to the **tibial tubercle/tuberosity**.
5. Ask the model to extend and flex the **knee joint**. Palpate the margins of the **ligamentum patellae** and borders of the **patella**.

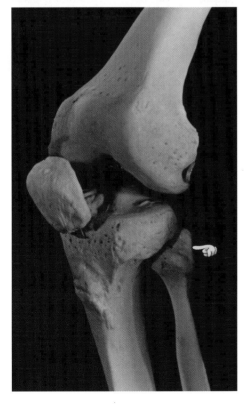

96. HEAD OF FIBULA

1. Ask the model to flex the **knee joint** against resistance.
2. Place the palmar surface of the index finger on the lateral aspect of the lower one-third of the **thigh**.
3. Palpate downwards towards the **lateral aspect of the knee joint** and identify the strong, rounded and distinct **tendon of biceps femoris muscle**.
4. Ask the model to rotate the **tibia** in a lateral direction to make the tendon more distinct.
5. Palpate the tendon to its major distal attachment, which is a prominent subcutaneous bony projection lying posterolateral to the **lateral condyle of tibia**.
6. This prominent bony projection lying 1 cm inferior to the **knee joint** is the **head of fibula**.

97. NECK OF FIBULA

1. Identify and palpate the **head of fibula** (*Objective No 96*).
2. Identify the **styloid process of the head of fibula** projecting upwards from the **posterior surface of the head of fibula**.
3. Identify the **tendon of biceps femoris** attaching to the **head of fibula**.
4. Palpate the **neck of fibula** located inferior to the **head of fibula**.
5. Note the subcutaneous position of the **common peroneal nerve** as it passes across the posterior aspect of the **head of fibula** and then forwards round the **neck of fibula**.

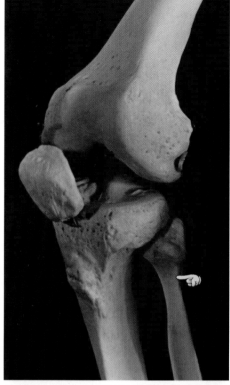

98. TIBIAL TUBEROSITY

1. Ask the model to sit down.
2. Identify the **borders of the patella** (*Objective No 95*) and **ligamentum patellae**.
3. Trace the **ligamentum patellae** from the **apex of the patella** (inferior pole) downwards to its attachment to the **tibial tuberosity**.
4. The **tibial tuberosity** can be palpated as a subcutaneous, prominent bony projection in the midline on the **shaft of tibia** immediately inferior to the anterior surface marking of the **knee joint**.

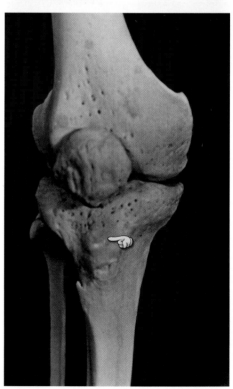

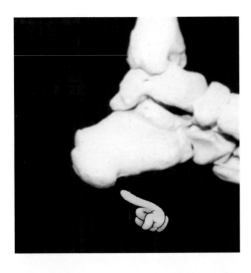

99. MEDIAL PROCESS OF CALCANEAL TUBEROSITY

1. Mark the inferior border of the **medial malleolus of tibia**.
2. Mark the position of the **sustentaculum tali**, inferior to the **medial malleolus of tibia**.
3. Palpate a point approximately 2.5 cm below the **sustentaculum tali** and move the palpating fingertip in a posterior direction for about 2.5 cm on the medial surface of the **calcaneus** and identify a firm bony prominence which is the **medial process of the calcaneal tuberosity**.

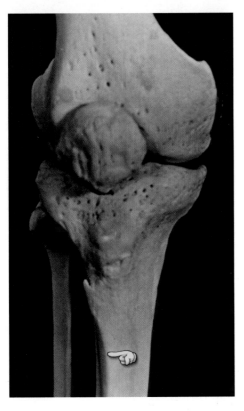

100. ANTERIOR BORDER OF THE SHAFT OF TIBIA

1. Palpate and mark the **tibial tuberosity** (*Objective No 98*).
2. Palpate and mark the sharp, sinuous, subcutaneous **anterior border of tibia** downwards towards the **ankle** region.
3. Note that as the **anterior border of tibia** approaches the lower extremity of the **shaft of tibia** it becomes covered by the **tendon of tibialis anterior**.
4. Note the smooth, flat, medial and subcutaneous **shaft of tibia** which merges with the **medial malleolus of tibia** below and the **medial condyle of tibia** above (*Objectives Nos 92 and 101*).

101. MEDIAL MALLEOLUS

1. Place the palpating fingertips on the anteromedial flat subcutaneous surface of the **shaft of tibia**.
2. Palpate towards the medial aspect of the foot and observe how the subcutaneous surface of the **shaft of tibia** becomes continuous below with a blunt, bony, visible prominence on the medial aspect of the ankle.
3. This visible bony prominence is the **medial malleolus of the tibia**.
4. Note that the **inferior border of the medial malleolus** is more anterior than the **lateral malleolus of the fibula**.
5. Note that the sharp, projecting, subcutaneous **lateral malleolus of the fibula** is more posterior and terminates approximately 1.5 cm below the **medial malleolus of the tibia**.

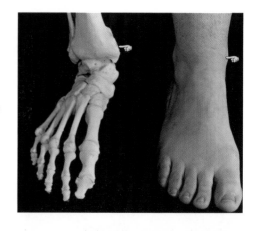

102. PERONEAL TUBERCLE

1. Mark the tip of the **lateral malleolus of fibula**.
2. Mark the base of the **5th metatarsal**.
3. Ask the model to evert the lateral border of the foot.
4. Identify the tendon of **peroneus brevis** passing round the lateral **malleolus of fibula** to its distal attachment on the base of the **5th metatarsal**.
5. Identify the tendon of **peroneus longus** passing round the lateral **malleolus of fibula** to the groove on the **cuboid**.
6. Palpate the lateral surface of the **calcaneus** and mark a point between the tendons of **peroneus brevis** and **peroneus longus** approximately 2.5 cm inferior to the tip of the **lateral malleolus of fibula**.
7. At this point a prominent bony process may be palpated on the lateral surface of the **calcaneus** approximately 2.5 cm proximal to the base of the **5th metatarsal**.
8. This prominent bony process is the **peroneal tubercle**.
9. The tendon of **peroneus brevis** passes above the **peroneal tubercle**.
10. The tendon of **peroneus longus** passes inferior to the **peroneal tubercle**.

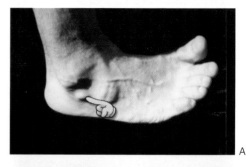
A

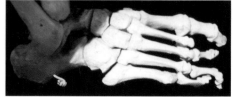
B

103. LATERAL MALLEOLUS

1. The sharp, pointed, bony, subcutaneous projection formed by the **lateral malleolus** can be observed on the lateral aspect of the **ankle**.
2. Identify the **medial malleolus** (*Objective No 101*).
3. Note how the **lateral malleolus of fibula** lies more posterior than the **medial malleolus of tibia**.
4. Note how the tip of the **lateral malleolus of fibula** descends to a level at least 1.5 cm below that of the **inferior border of the medial malleolus of tibia**.

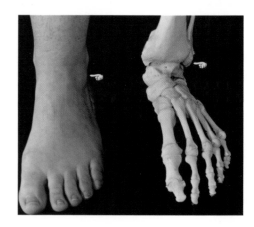

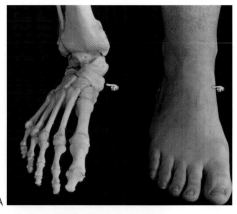

A

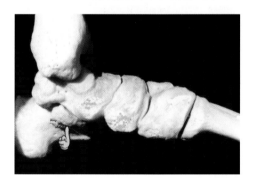

B

104. TUBEROSITY OF NAVICULAR

1. Identify the **sustentaculum tali** (*Objective No 105*).
2. Maintain the **foot** in the anatomical position.
3. Move the tip of the index finger forwards from the **sustentaculum tali** approximately 2 cm in the same horizontal plane.
4. A prominent, subcutaneous, raised bony projection can be felt at this point.
5. This prominent projection is the **tuberosity of navicular**.
6. On applying maximal resistance to the movement of inversion, the prominent tendon of **tibialis posterior** is observed passing to the **tuberosity of navicular** from the region of the **medial malleolus** and superior to the **sustentaculum tali**.

105. SUSTENTACULUM TALI

1. Keeping the **foot** in the anatomical position, place the tip of the index finger on the **medial border of the foot**.
2. The tip of the index finger should point towards the **inferior border of the medial malleolus of tibia**.
3. Palpate with firm pressure from the **medial border of the foot** in an upwards direction towards the **inferior border of the medial malleolus**.
4. Approximately 2 cm below the inferior border of the **medial malleolus** a projecting shelf of bone is encountered by the palpating fingertip.
5. This projecting shelf of bone is the **sustentaculum tali**.

106. HEAD AND NECK OF TALUS

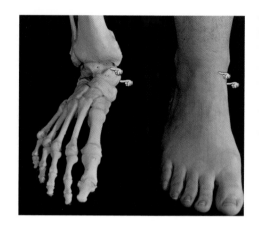

1. Identify and palpate the **medial malleolus of tibia** (*Objective No 101*).
2. Identify and mark the depression, which lies below the line of direction taken by the **tendon of tibialis anterior** when the ankle joint is dorsiflexed and the **foot** inverted against resistance.
3. The **tuberosity of navicular** (*Objective No 104*) can be palpated 2 cm inferior and anterior to the **medial malleolus**.
4. A line drawn on the **medial aspect of the foot** from the inferior border of the **medial malleolus** to the **tuberosity of navicular** with a slight upwards convexity crosses the **head of talus**.
5. The **head of talus** can be identified at the midpoint with the **neck of talus** placed proximal to the **head of talus**.
6. Passively invert the foot. The superior and lateral aspects of the **head** and **neck of talus** can be identified and palpated 3 cm anterior to the **lateral malleolus of fibula** on the lateral aspect of the foot.

107. CUBOID BONE

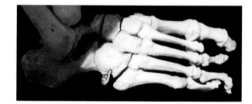

1. Identify the **lateral border of the foot**.
2. Mark a point halfway between the tip of the **little toe** and the posterior border of the **calcaneus** on the **lateral border of the foot**.
3. Identify the prominent tubercle on the base of the **5th metatarsal bone**.
4. Grasp the base of the **5th metatarsal** between the tip of the index finger and thumb and note the gliding action at the joint between the **4th** and **5th metatarsal bones** when they are moved.
5. Proximal to the base of the **4th** and **5th metatarsals** lies the **cuboid bone**.
6. Placing the thumb tip on the **cuboid** and tip of the index finger underneath the **cuboid**, hold the bone firmly.
7. With the other index finger and thumb grasp the base of the **4th** and **5th metatarsals** and note the sliding action when they are moved against the **cuboid**.
8. Evert the **foot** against maximal resistance and note the **tendon of peroneus brevis** as it passes to the base of the **5th metatarsal bone**.
9. The **tendon of peroneus brevis** passes over the **cuboid bone**.
10. The **tendon of peroneus longus** passes under and grooves the **cuboid bone** immediately proximal to the base of the **5th metatarsal bone**.

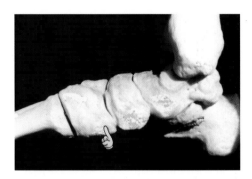

108. MEDIAL CUNEIFORM BONE

1. Identify the **tuberosity of navicular** (*Objective No 104*).
2. Note the **tendon of tibialis posterior** passing to its principal distal attachment, the **tuberosity of navicular**, when the **ankle joint** is plantarflexed and the **foot** is inverted against resistance.
3. Dorsiflex the **ankle joint** and invert the **foot** against resistance.
4. A thick distinct tendon can be observed and palpated passing distal to the **tuberosity of navicular** on the **medial side of the foot**. This is the **tendon of tibialis anterior**.
5. The **tendon of tibialis anterior** attaches to the **medial cuneiform** and base of the **1st metatarsal bone**.
6. The **medial cuneiform bone** can be palpated at this point.

109. BASE OF THE 5TH METATARSAL BONE OF THE FOOT

1. Identify and palpate the **lateral border of the foot** from the **calcaneus** posteriorly to the tip of the **distal phalanx of the 5th toe**.
2. The base of the **5th metatarsal bone** is located halfway along the **lateral border of the foot** where it may be palpated as a prominent bony feature.
3. When the **lateral border of the foot** is raised in eversion against maximal resistance, the **tendon of peroneus brevis** may be identified (*Objective No 140*) passing round the **lateral malleolus of the fibula** to the base of the **5th metatarsal**.

Joints of the Lower Limb

110. SACROILIAC

1. Identify and mark the position of the **posterior superior iliac spines** which are overlaid by two dimples (*Objective No 86*).
2. The **posterior superior iliac spine** is positioned over the centre of the **sacroiliac joint**.

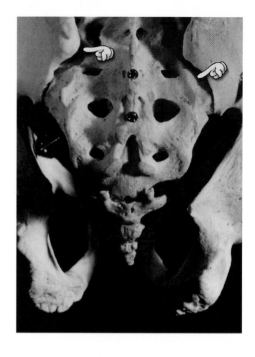

111. HIP (ANTERIOR SURFACE MARKING OF MIDPOINT)

1. Identify the **anterior superior iliac spine** and surface mark (*Objective No 86*).
2. Explain the technique and ask the model to self-identify the position of the **symphysis pubis**.
3. Draw an imaginary line from the **anterior superior iliac spine** to the indicated position of the **symphysis pubis**.
4. Identify the midpoint of the imagined line.
5. The anterior surface marking of the centre of the **hip joint** lies approximately 2 cm inferior to the midpoint of the above line.

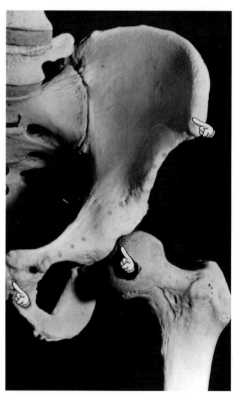

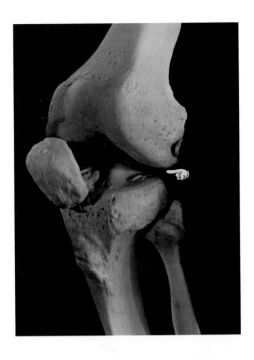

112. KNEE

1. Ask the model to sit down.
2. Identify the **head of fibula** (*Objective No 96*).
3. The line of the **knee joint** lies 1 cm superior to the **head of fibula**.
4. Identify the bony edge of the **tibial plateau** of the **lateral tibial condyle** forming the inferior boundary of the **anterolateral** compartment of the **knee joint** (*Objective No 94*).
5. Palpate the line of the **knee joint** towards the anterior midline over the **ligamentum patellae** to the **anteromedial** compartment lying between the **medial condyle of femur** and the **medial condyle of tibia**.
6. Identify the bony edge of the **tibial plateau** of the **medial condyle of tibia**.
7. Project an imagined line round the medial, posterior and lateral aspects of the **knee** crossing ligaments, muscles and tendons.

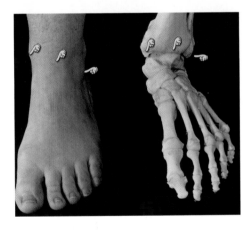

113. ANKLE

1. Palpate the **lateral malleolus of fibula** (*Objective No 103*).
2. Note that the tip of the **lateral malleolus of fibula** projects approximately 1.5 cm below the **medial malleolus of tibia** and lies on a more posterior plane.
3. Palpate the **medial malleolus of tibia** (*Objective No 101*).
4. Note that the **medial malleolus of tibia** forms a blunt, visible subcutaneous prominence on the **medial aspect of the ankle** and lies on a more anterior plane than the **lateral malleolus of fibula**. The inferior edge of the **medial malleolus** lies approximately 1.5 cm above the tip of the **lateral malleolus**.
5. Note that the **anterior and inferior edges** of the **shaft of tibia** adjacent to the **medial malleolus** can be palpated.
6. Mark a point 2 cm above the tip of the **lateral malleolus** and mark a second point 1 cm above the inferior border of the **medial malleolus**; join both points.
7. This line represents the horizontal component of the **ankle joint**.
8. Support the **foot** and passively **plantar- and dorsiflex the ankle joint**. Palpate along the anterior and inferior edges of the **shaft of tibia** adjacent to the **medial malleolus of tibia**. Palpate and detect the joint line.
9. Tendons crossing the anterior aspect of the **ankle joint** obscure the remaining joint line.

114. TARSOMETATARSAL

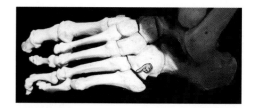

1. Identify and mark the outline of the **cuboid bone** (*Objective No 107*).
2. Identify and mark the base of the **5th metatarsal bone** (*Objective No 109*).
3. Grasp the **cuboid bone** between the tip of the index finger on the dorsal surface and the thumb tip below on the plantar surface.
4. With the tip of the other index finger placed on the top of the base of the **5th metatarsal** and the other thumb placed below on the plantar surface, grasp the bone firmly.
5. Produce a transverse gliding action between the **cuboid** and the base of the **5th metatarsal bone**.
6. The gliding movement takes place at the **5th tarsometatarsal joint**.

115. METATARSOPHALANGEAL

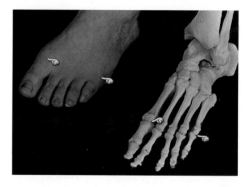

1. Identify and mark the base of the **5th metatarsal bone** (*Objective No 109*).
2. Palpate the base, move distally along the shaft and identify the neck and head of the **5th metatarsal bone**.
3. Fully flex the **5th toe** keeping a fingertip on the **head of the metatarsal bone**.
4. Extend and flex the **5th toe** and note the position where movement takes place immediately distal to the **head of the 5th metatarsal bone**.
5. Mark the position where movement between the **head of the 5th metatarsal bone** and the **base of the proximal phalanx of the 5th toe** takes place with a line to indicate the joint space.

9

Muscles of the Lower Limb

116. ILIOPSOAS

1. Ask the model to assume a position of supine lying with comfortable support to fix the starting position and reduce muscle tone in the **abdominal muscles**.
2. Passively flex the **hip** and **knee joints** to 90° and support manually.
3. Apply maximal resistance to the anterior surface of the **thigh** and ask the model to flex the **hip joint**.
4. Palpate the **iliopsoas** as it passes over the anterior surface of the **hip joint** to its distal attachment on the **lesser trochanter** and **shaft of femur**.

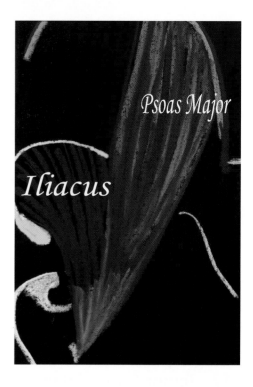

117. TENSOR FASCIAE LATAE

1. Surface mark the **greater trochanter of femur** (*Objective No 87*).
2. Ask the model to flex and abduct the **hip joint** against maximal resistance.
3. The **muscle belly of tensor fasciae latae** can be palpated approximately 5 cm anterior to the surface marking of the **greater trochanter of femur**.
4. Observe the fibres passing down the **anterolateral aspect of the thigh** to assist in the formation of the **iliotibial tract**.

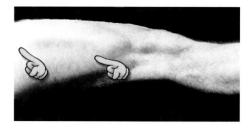

118. VASTUS MEDIALIS

1. Ask the model to sit down and fully extend the **knee joint** against maximal resistance.
2. **Vastus medialis** functions as a member of the quadriceps group during extension of the **knee joint**.
3. **Vastus medialis** can be palpated on the anteromedial aspect of the **thigh** medial to **rectus femoris** and fibres identified passing to their distal attachment on the medial aspect of the **patella**, quadriceps expansion and indirectly to the **tibial tuberosity** through the **ligamentum patellae**.

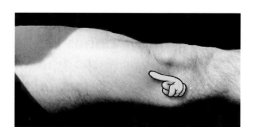

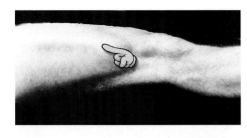

119. VASTUS LATERALIS

1. Ask the model to sit down and fully extend the **knee joint** against maximal resistance.
2. **Vastus lateralis** functions as a member of the quadriceps group during extension of the **knee joint**.
3. **Vastus lateralis** can be palpated on the anterolateral aspect of the **thigh**, lateral to **rectus femoris** and fibres identified passing to their distal attachment on the lateral aspect of the **patella**, quadriceps expansion and indirectly to the **tibial tuberosity** through the **ligamentum patellae**.

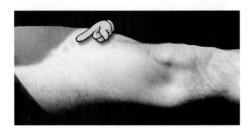

120. VASTUS INTERMEDIUS

1. Ask the model to sit down and fully extend the **knee joint** against maximal resistance.
2. **Vastus intermedius** functions as a member of the quadriceps group during extension of the **knee joint**.
3. **Vastus intermedius muscle fibres** cannot be palpated as they are deep to the **rectus femoris muscle**.
4. The **quadriceps femoris tendon** is formed by the unification of the **three vasti muscles** and **rectus femoris**.
5. The **patella**, a sesamoid bone developed within the **quadriceps femoris tendon**, improves the mechanical advantage by altering the angle of pull of the **quadriceps femoris group** during extension of the **knee joint**.

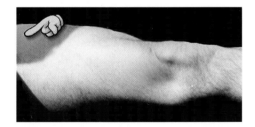

121. RECTUS FEMORIS

1. Surface mark the **anterior inferior iliac spine**, projected position of the superior edge of the **acetabulum**, **base of patella** and **tuberosity of tibia**.
2. Ask the model to sit down.
3. Ask the model to flex the **hip joint** a few degrees and fully extend the **knee joint** against maximal resistance.
4. The **rectus femoris** may be palpated passing across the anterior aspect of the **thigh** from its proximal attachments on the **innominate bone** to its distal attachment on the **base of patella** and finally by the **ligamentum patellae** to the **tuberosity of tibia**.

122. GROUP ACTION OF HIP JOINT ROTATORS

1. The obturator externus, obturator internus, gemellus superior, gemellus inferior, quadratus femoris and piriformis muscles surround and stabilise the **head of femur** in the **acetabulum** of the **innominate bone** as they pass to their distal attachments on the medial and posterior surfaces of the **greater trochanter**.
2. Ask the model to rotate the **hip joint** in a lateral direction against maximal resistance to demonstrate the group action of the above muscles.
3. With the exception of **piriformis** they cannot be palpated.

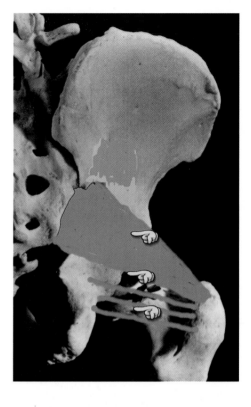

123. PIRIFORMIS

1. Ask the model to take up a position of prone lying with support to reduce muscle tone.
2. Surface mark the **posterior superior iliac spine**, upper border of the **greater trochanter** and **tip of the coccyx**.
3. Draw a vertical line between the **tip of the coccyx** and the **posterior superior iliac spine**. Mark the midpoint.
4. Draw a line from the midpoint to the upper border of the **greater trochanter**.
5. The line in step 4 marks the inferior border of **piriformis**.
6. Ask the model to rotate the **hip joint** in a lateral direction against maximal resistance to demonstrate the action of **piriformis**.

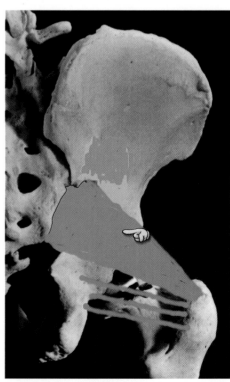

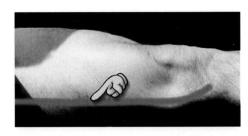

124. GRACILIS

1. Ask the model to take up a supine position to reduce muscle tone.
2. Ask the model to slightly flex and strongly adduct the **hip joint** against maximal resistance.
3. Palpate **gracilis** on the medial aspect of the **thigh**, anterior to **semitendinosus** and trace the fibres as it passes to its distal attachment on the medial surface of the **shaft of tibia** immediately inferior to the **condyle of tibia**.

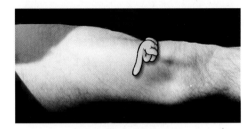

125. ADDUCTOR MAGNUS

1. Ask the model to take up a position of supine lying with support to reduce muscle tone.
2. Surface mark the **adductor tubercle** (*Objective No 91*).
3. Ask the model to slightly extend and adduct the **hip joint** against maximal resistance.
4. Palpate the fibres of **adductor magnus** on the medial surface of the middle part of the **thigh** as they pass to the **shaft of femur** and **adductor tubercle** on the **medial condyle of femur**.

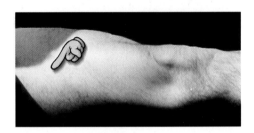

126. ADDUCTOR LONGUS

1. Ask the model to take up a position of supine lying with support to reduce muscle tone.
2. Ask the model to slightly flex and strongly adduct the **hip joint** against maximal resistance.
3. Palpate the **muscle fibres of adductor longus** on the medial aspect of the upper one-third of the **thigh** lateral to **gracilis**.

127. PECTINEUS AND ADDUCTOR BREVIS

Pectineus
1. Ask the model to take up a supine position to reduce muscle tone.
2. Ask the model to slightly flex and adduct the **hip joint** against maximal resistance.
3. The muscle fibres of **pectineus** can be palpated lateral to **adductor longus** as the fibres pass from the **pubis** to their distal attachment below the **lesser trochanter of femur**.

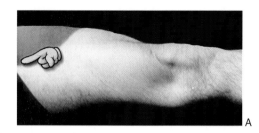

A

Adductor brevis
1. Ask the model to take up a position of supine lying with support to reduce muscle tone.
2. Ask the model to slightly flex and adduct the **hip joint** against maximal resistance.
3. **Adductor brevis** passes from the **ramus of pubis** to its distal attachment on the **shaft of femur** immediately below the **lesser trochanter** and is difficult to palpate without causing discomfort to the model.

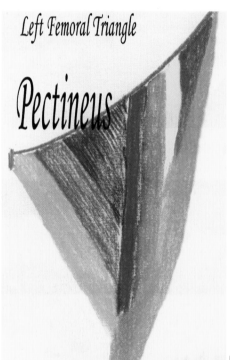

Left Femoral Triangle

Pectineus

B

128. GLUTEUS MAXIMUS

1. Ask the model to take up the position of prone lying with one **knee joint** flexed to 90°.
2. Apply maximal resistance to the posterior surface of the **thigh**.
3. Ask the model to extend the **hip joint** against maximal resistance with the **knee joint** flexed to 90°.
4. The contracting fibres of **gluteus maximus** can be observed and palpated as a distinct rounded muscular contour forming the **buttock** on the posterior aspect of the **hip**.
5. Ask the model to sit down and place the fingertips on the **ischial tuberosities**.
6. Ask the model to rise from the position of sitting to standing with the fingertips on the **ischial tuberosities**.
7. **Gluteus maximus** passes over and covers the **ischial tuberosities** as the model takes up the standing position and pushes the palpating fingertips from the **ischial tuberosities**.

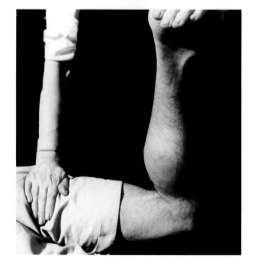

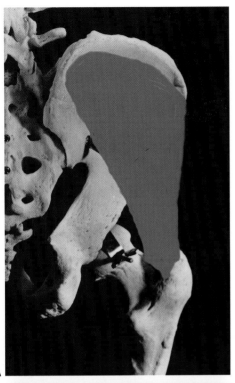

A

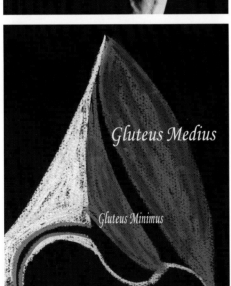

Gluteus Medius

Gluteus Minimus

B

129. GLUTEUS MEDIUS

1. Ask the model to weight bear on one **foot** and maintain the pelvis level with the **anterior superior iliac spines** (*Objective No 86*) in the same horizontal plane.
2. The **muscle belly of gluteus medius** can be palpated on the weight-bearing **lower limb** 5 cm superior to the **greater trochanter of femur** (*Objective No 87*) as it contracts to maintain the pelvis level, working with **quadratus lumborum** (*Objective No 181*) of the opposite side.
3. Ask the model to take up a position of supine lying.
4. Ask the model to abduct and medially rotate the **hip joint** against maximal resistance.
5. The **muscle belly of gluteus medius** can be palpated 5 cm superior to the **greater trochanter** when this is abducted against maximal resistance.

130. GLUTEUS MINIMUS

1. Ask the model to take up the position of prone lying with one **knee joint** flexed to 90°.
2. Ask the model to medially rotate and abduct the **hip joint** against maximal resistance.
3. The muscle fibres of **gluteus minimus** are mainly overlaid by the fibres of **gluteus medius**.
4. Palpate approximately 5 cm superior to the **greater trochanter of femur** (*Objective No 87*) and move slightly forward to a position anterior to the contraction of **gluteus medius**.

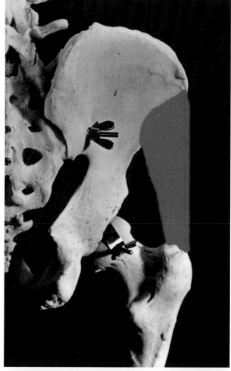

A

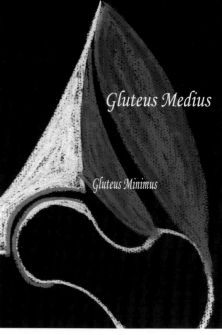

Gluteus Medius

Gluteus Minimus

B

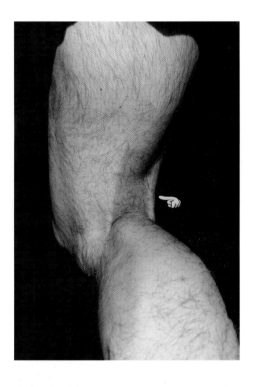

131. BICEPS FEMORIS

1. Surface mark the **head of fibula** (*Objective No 96*) and **lateral condyle of tibia**.
2. Ask the model to flex and laterally rotate the **knee joint** against maximal resistance.
3. Observe and palpate the long thick tendon on the lateral aspect of the **popliteal fossa** passing to its major distal attachment on the **head of fibula** and minor attachment on the **lateral condyle of tibia**.

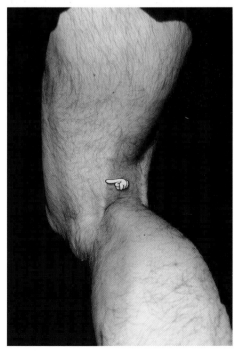

132. SEMITENDINOSUS

1. Surface mark the medial surface of the upper quarter of the **shaft of tibia** and adjacent surface of the **medial condyle of tibia**.
2. Ask the model to flex and medially rotate the **knee joint** against maximal resistance.
3. Observe and palpate the long thin tendon of **semitendinosus** on the medial side of the **popliteal fossa**, lying posterior and superficial to the **semimembranosus** as it passes to its distal attachment on the upper and medial surface of the **shaft of tibia** and adjacent **medial condyle of tibia**.

133. SEMIMEMBRANOSUS

1. Surface mark the posterior surface of the **medial condyle of tibia**.
2. Ask the model to flex the **knee joint** to ninety degrees and medially rotate the **tibia** against maximal resistance.
3. Palpate the long thin **tendon of semitendinosus** passing to the medial aspect of the **medial condyle of tibia**.
4. Palpate on each side of the tendon of **semitendinosus**, the tendon of **semimembranosus** placed deep and anterior to the **semitendinosus**.
5. The **tendon of semimembranosus** lies deep to the **tendons of gracilis** and **semitendinosus** at the level of the **knee joint** as it passes to its distal attachment on the posterior surface of the **medial condyle of tibia**.

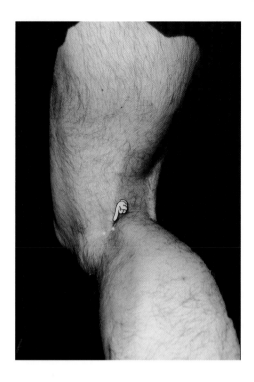

134. SARTORIUS

1. Surface mark the **anterior superior iliac spine**.
2. Surface mark the **medial condyle of tibia**.
3. Ask the model to take up the position of 'tailor sitting', i.e. the **hip joints** flexed and in lateral rotation, the **knee joints** flexed and the feet crossed.
4. Apply maximal resistance to the medial surface of the **medial condyle of tibia** and ask the model to flex the **knee joint**, then medially rotate and flex the **hip joint** against resistance applied to the medial aspect of the **medial condyle of tibia**.
5. Palpate **sartorius** from its proximal attachment to the **anterior superior iliac spine** and adjacent bone, down and across the **thigh** to its distal attachment on the anterior and medial surface of the **medial condyle of tibia**.

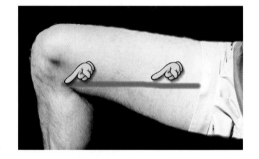

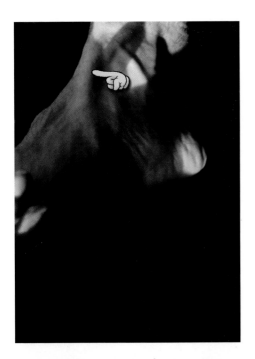

135. TIBIALIS ANTERIOR

1. Ask the model to sit down.
2. Surface mark the **lateral condyle of tibia**, **medial malleolus**, base of the **1st metatarsal** and **medial cuneiform**.
3. Ask the model to dorsiflex the **ankle joint** and invert and adduct the **tarsal joints** against maximal resistance.
4. Palpate the **muscle belly of tibialis anterior** lateral to the **anterior border of tibia** in the upper two-thirds of the **leg**.
5. Observe and palpate the **tendon of tibialis anterior** as it passes in the lower one-third of the **leg** to the medial side, anterior to the **medial malleolus** to its distal attachment on the plantar surface of the base of the **1st metatarsal bone** and medial surface of the **medial cuneiform**.

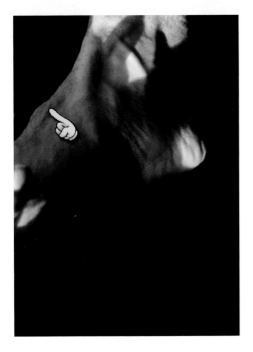

136. EXTENSOR HALLUCIS LONGUS

1. Ask the model to sit down.
2. Surface mark the dorsal surface of the base of the **distal phalanx of the hallux (big toe)**.
3. Ask the model to dorsiflex the **ankle joint** and fully extend the **interphalangeal joints of the hallux** against maximal resistance.
4. Observe and palpate the distinct **tendon of extensor hallucis longus** as it becomes subcutaneous in the lower one-third of the **leg** and passes slightly medially across the dorsum of the **foot** towards its distal attachment on the dorsal surface of the base of the **distal phalanx of the hallux (big toe)**.

137. EXTENSOR HALLUCIS BREVIS

1. Ask the model to sit down.
2. Ask the model to extend the **toes** against maximal resistance.
3. Palpate the **muscle belly of extensor digitorum brevis** and the four tendons passing to the **medial four toes**.
4. Identify the **tendon of extensor hallucis brevis** on the lateral side of the **tendon of extensor hallucis longus** as it passes to its distal attachment on the base of the **proximal phalanx of the 1st toe**.
5. The muscle fibres and **tendon of extensor hallucis brevis** cross the **dorsalis pedis artery**.

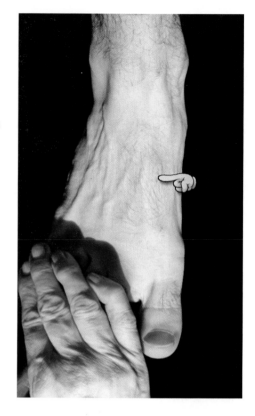

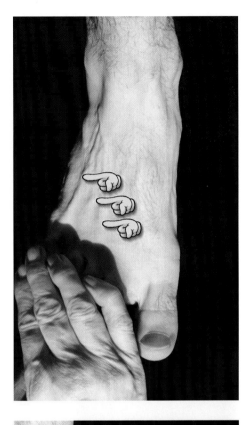

138. EXTENSOR DIGITORUM LONGUS

1. Ask the model to sit down.
2. Ask the model to dorsiflex the **ankle joint** and to fully extend the **interphalangeal joints** of the **lateral four toes** against maximal resistance.
3. Observe and palpate the **tendon of extensor digitorum longus** as it crosses the anterior aspect of the **ankle joint** and **dorsum of the foot** where it divides into four distinct tendons, each passing to its distal attachment on the dorsal surface of the **middle and distal phalanges** of the **lateral four toes**.

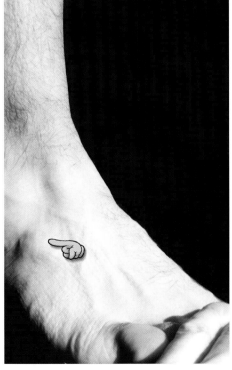

139. EXTENSOR DIGITORUM BREVIS

1. Ask the model to sit down.
2. Ask the model to dorsiflex the **ankle joint** and extend the **interphalangeal joints** of the **lateral four toes** against maximal resistance.
3. On the **dorsum of the foot** lateral to the **tendon of extensor digitorum longus** passing to its distal attachment on the **little toe**, the **muscle belly of extensor digitorum brevis** can be observed and palpated.
4. Palpate the **muscle belly of extensor digitorum brevis** on the **dorsum of the foot** approximately 5 cm distal to the **anterior border of the lateral malleolus**.

140. PERONEUS BREVIS

1. Ask the model to sit down.
2. Ask the model to plantarflex the **ankle joint** and evert the **tarsal joints** against maximal resistance applied to the lateral border of the **foot**.
3. Surface mark the **lateral malleolus** and base of the **5th metatarsal bone**.
4. Surface mark the position of the **peroneal trochlea** on the lateral surface of the **calcaneum**.
5. Observe and palpate the **muscle belly of peroneus brevis** arising from the lateral surface of the lower two-thirds of the **shaft of fibula** and the tendon passing close to the posterior border of the **lateral malleolus**, round and inferior to the **peroneal trochlea** to its distal attachment on the **tuberosity of the base of the 5th metatarsal bone**.

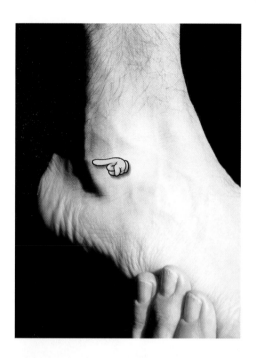

141. PERONEUS LONGUS

1. Ask the model to **plantarflex** the **ankle joint**, and evert and abduct the **tarsal joints** against maximal resistance applied to the **lateral border of the foot**.
2. Surface mark the **head of fibula, lateral condyle of tibia, lateral malleolus**, base of the **5th metatarsal bone, groove on cuboid** and **medial cuneiform**.
3. Palpate the **muscle belly of peroneus longus** in the lateral compartment, upper one-third of the **leg** anterior to **soleus**.
4. Palpate the **tendon of peroneus longus** immediately posterior to the **peroneus brevis tendon** and posterior border of the **lateral malleolus of fibula** as it passes down and round the **peroneal trochlea** to reach the **groove on cuboid** and on to its distal attachment on the lateral margin of the plantar surface of the **medial cuneiform** and base of the **1st metatarsal bone**.

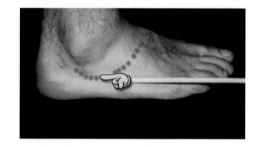

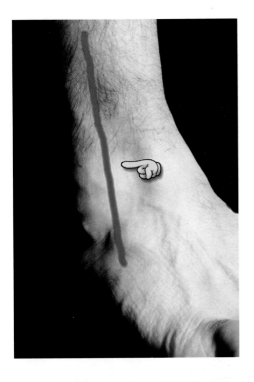

142. PERONEUS TERTIUS

1. Ask the model to dorsiflex the **ankle joint**, and evert and abduct the **tarsal joints** against maximal resistance applied to the dorsal surface of the base of the **5th metatarsal**.
2. Palpate the **muscle belly of peroneus tertius** on the anterior surface of the lower **one-third of the fibula**.
3. Palpate the tendon proximal to the dorsal surface of the base of the **5th metatarsal**.

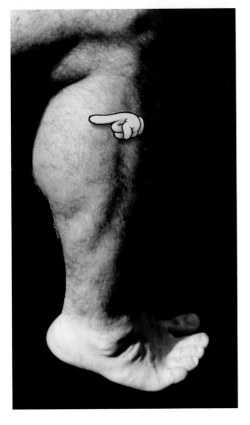

143. GASTROCNEMIUS

1. Surface mark the popliteal space.
2. Ask the model to plantarflex the **ankle joint** against maximal resistance as in the action of walking up stairs.
3. Palpate the **subcutaneous medial** and **lateral heads of gastrocnemius** forming the distinct lower boundaries of the **popliteal space** as far down as the middle of the **calf** where they fuse to form the **tendocalcaneus**.
4. The **tendocalcaneus** can be observed and palpated as it passes to its distal attachment on the **posterior surface of the calcaneus**.

144. SOLEUS

1. Ask the model to sit down with the **knee joint** flexed to 90°.
2. Ask the model to raise the heel against maximal resistance.
3. Observe and palpate the lateral border of **soleus** anterior to the **lateral head of gastrocnemius** and inferior to the **head and neck of fibula**.
4. The **soleus** is placed anterior to the **gastrocnemius** but is exposed on the lateral aspect of the lower part of the **leg** where it can be observed and palpated.
5. The **soleus**, which is a postural muscle, assists **gastrocnemius** in forming the **tendocalcaneus** as it passes to its distal attachment on the posterior surface of the **calcaneus**.

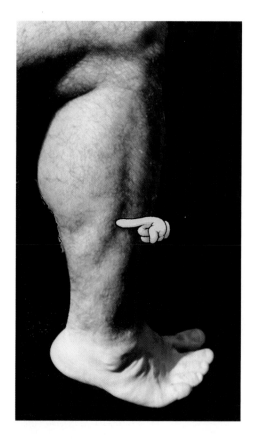

145. POPLITEUS

1. Ask the model to walk forward two paces from the anatomical position.
2. The **popliteus muscle** unlocks the **knee joint** at the start of flexion which occurs in the first phase of walking when taking a step forwards with the non-weight-bearing **lower limb**.
3. The **muscle belly of popliteus** cannot be palpated as it lies deep to the **medial** and **lateral heads of gastrocnemius**.

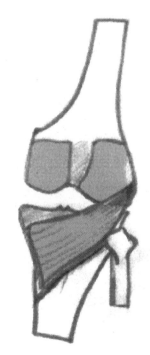

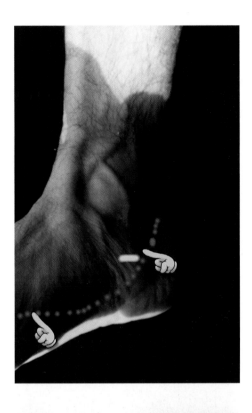

146. FLEXOR HALLUCIS LONGUS

1. Ask the model to take up a position of supine lying.
2. Ask the model to plantarflex the **ankle joint**, invert the **tarsal joints** and flex the **interphalangeal joints of the big toe** against maximal resistance.
3. Surface mark the **medial malleolus, sustentaculum tali** and the medial edge of the **calcaneal tendon**.
4. Palpate on a curved line from the medial border of the **calcaneal tendon** to the inferior border of the **sustentaculum tali** to identify the position of the **tendon of flexor hallucis longus**.
5. Palpate the plantar surface of the base of the **distal phalanx of the great toe** to identify the distal attachment of **flexor hallucis longus**.

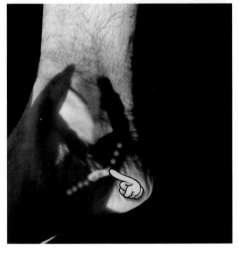

147. FLEXOR DIGITORUM LONGUS

1. Ask the model to take up a position of supine lying.
2. Ask the model to plantarflex the **ankle joint**, invert and adduct the **tarsal joint** and flex the **interphalangeal joints** of the **outer four toes** against maximal resistance.
3. Surface mark the position of the **sustentaculum tali**.
4. Palpate the medial surface of the **sustentaculum tali** and the plantar surface of the base of the **distal phalanx of the four outer toes** to identify the **tendon(s) of flexor digitorum longus**.

148. TIBIALIS POSTERIOR

1. Ask the model to take up a position of supine lying.
2. Ask the model to plantarflex the **ankle joint**, and invert and adduct the **tarsal joints** against maximal resistance.
3. Surface mark the **medial malleolus**, **sustentaculum tali** and **tuberosity of navicular**.
4. Observe and palpate the **tendon of tibialis posterior** as it passes round the posterior border of the **medial malleolus**, superior to the **sustentaculum tali** and to one of its principal distal attachments, the **tuberosity of the navicular bone**.

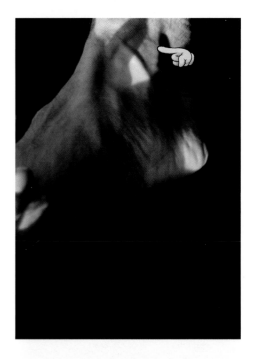

149. DORSAL INTEROSSEI

1. Ask the model to sit down and place one **foot** on a flat support (e.g. a book) with the joint line of the **metatarsophalangeal joints** on the edge of the book, **toes** parallel to the floor.
2. Ask the model to flex the **metatarsophalangeal joints** and extend the **interphalangeal joints of the toes**.
3. Ask the model to abduct the **middle toe** away from the side of the **2nd toe**, away from the midline passing through the **2nd toe**.

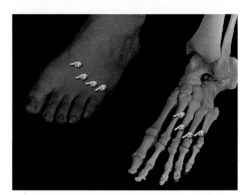

150. PLANTAR INTEROSSEI

1. Ask the model to sit down and place one **foot** on a flat support (e.g. a book) with the joint line of the **metatarsophalangeal joints** on the edge of the book, **toes** parallel to the floor.
2. Ask the model to flex the **metatarsophalangeal joints** and extend the **interphalangeal joints of the toes**.
3. Ask the model to maintain the position in step 2 and adduct the **little toe** against the lateral side of the **4th toe** and towards the midline passing through the **2nd toe**.

10

Superficial Veins of the Lower Limb

151. GREAT/LONG SAPHENOUS

1. Draw an oval on the medial aspect of the **thigh** immediately inferior to the medial attachment of the **inguinal ligament**.
2. Imagine a line drawn from the **anterior superior iliac spine** (*Objective No 86*) to the lateral edge of the **symphysis pubis**. This line is gently convex downwards.
3. Identify and mark the position of the **dorsal venous network** on the **dorsum** of the **foot**.
4. Identify and mark the position of the **medial malleolus of tibia** (*Objective No 101*).
5. Identify and mark the **adductor tubercle of femur** (*Objective No 91*).
6. Draw a line on the skin from the medial aspect of the **dorsal venous network**, passing anterior to the **medial malleolus**, ascending on the medial border of **soleus** (*Objective No 144*), crossing the **knee joint**, ascending the **thigh** on the medial aspect in the region of the **adductor tubercle** to reach the **saphenous opening** (step 1) to pierce fascia to join the **femoral vein**.
7. The **great/long saphenous vein** is often visible as it ascends anterior to the **medial malleolus**.

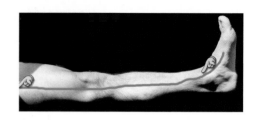

152. SMALL/SHORT SAPHENOUS

1. Identify and mark the position of the **dorsal venous network** in the **foot**.
2. Identify and mark the **lateral malleolus of fibula** (*Objective No 103*).
3. Identify and mark the **tendocalcaneus** (*Objectives Nos 143 and 144*).
4. Identify and mark the boundaries of the **popliteal fossa**.
5. Mark the midpoint of the **popliteal fossa**.
6. Draw a line from the lateral aspect of the **dorsal venous network**, posterior to the **lateral malleolus of fibula**, ascending to cross the **tendocalcaneus** to the midline.
7. Continue the line between the **medial** and **lateral heads of gastrocnemius** (*Objectives Nos 143 and 144*) to the midpoint of the **popliteal fossa**.
8. This line marks the course of the **short saphenous vein** from the lateral aspect of the **dorsal venous network** to the **popliteal fossa** where it pierces fascia to join the **popliteal vein**.

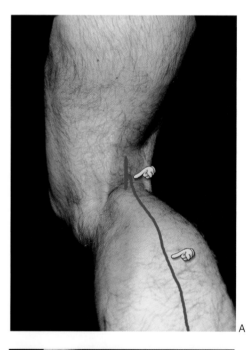

A

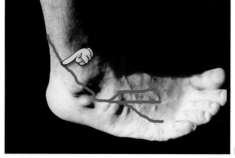

B

11

Arterial Pulses of the Lower Limb

153. FEMORAL PULSE

1. Ask the model to abduct, flex and laterally rotate the **hip joint**.
2. Identify and mark the **anterior superior iliac spine** (*Objective No 86*).
3. Ask the model to place a fingertip on the **symphysis pubis**.
4. Draw a line from the **anterior superior iliac spine** in the direction of the **symphysis pubis**.
5. Mark a point on the line midway between the **anterior superior iliac spine** and the **symphysis pubis**.
6. At this point identify and count the pulse of the **femoral artery** as it crosses the **ramus of pubis** and the anterior surface of the **head of femur**.

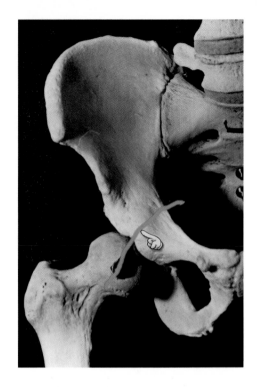

154. POPLITEAL PULSE

1. Ask the model to sit down.
2. Identify and mark the **adductor tubercle of femur** (*Objective No 91*).
3. Draw a line from a point immediately superior to the **adductor tubercle of femur** to the midpoint of a line on the posterior surface of the **knee joint** (*Objective No 112*) joining the **medial** and **lateral condyles of femur**.
4. The pulse of the **popliteal artery** can be identified and counted on the midpoint or slightly medial to the midpoint of the line joining the **medial** and **lateral condyles of femur**.

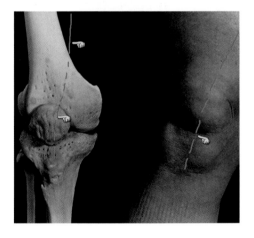

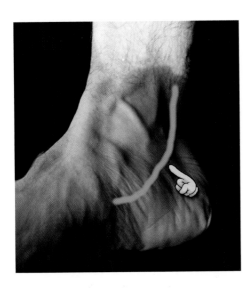

155. POSTERIOR TIBIAL PULSE

1. Identify and mark the **medial malleolus of tibia** (*Objective No 101*).
2. Identify and mark the **sustentaculum tali** (*Objective No 105*).
3. Draw a line from a point posterior to the **medial malleolus** passing inferior to the **sustentaculum tali**.
4. The pulse of the **posterior tibial artery** can be identified and counted midway between the tip of the **medial malleolus of tibia** and the **medial tubercle of calcaneum**.

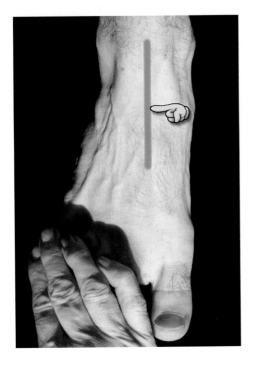

156. DORSALIS PEDIS PULSE

1. Identify and surface mark the **ankle joint** (*Objective No 113*).
2. Ask the model to extend the **big toe** against resistance.
3. Identify and mark the **tendon of extensor hallucis longus** (*Objective No 136*).
4. Identify the **dorsalis pedis artery** lying lateral to the **tendon of extensor hallucis longus** on the **dorsum of the foot**.
5. Count the pulse of the **dorsalis pedis artery**.

12

Peripheral Nerves of the Lower Limb

157. SCIATIC NERVE UNDER GLUTEUS MAXIMUS

1. Surface mark the **posterior superior iliac spine** (*Objective No 86*).
2. Surface mark the position of the **ischial tuberosity** (*Objective No 88*).
3. Surface mark the position of the **greater trochanter** (*Objective No 87*).
4. Draw a vertical line connecting the **posterior superior iliac spine** and the **ischial tuberosity**.
5. Mark the midpoint of the vertical line and a point just lateral to the midpoint.
6. Draw a horizontal line from the **ischial tuberosity** to the **greater trochanter**.
7. Mark the midpoint of the horizontal line and a point just medial to the midpoint.
8. Join the lateral point in step 5 to the medial point in step 7 with a line presenting a gradual convexity towards the lateral aspect.
9. Continue to draw the line in a vertical direction down towards the apex of the **popliteal fossa**.
10. The line drawn represents the course of the **sciatic nerve** which splits into the **common peroneal and tibial nerves** during its descent to the **popliteal fossa**.

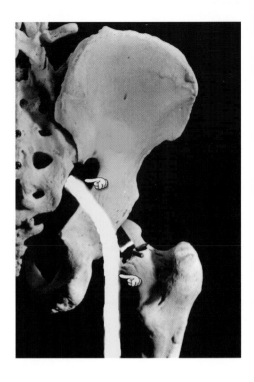

158. COMMON PERONEAL NERVE IN THE REGION OF THE KNEE JOINT

1. Ask the model to flex the **knee joint** to a right angle.
2. Mark the boundaries of the **popliteal fossa**.
3. Identify the **tendon of biceps femoris** (*Objective No 131*).
4. Mark the **apex of the popliteal fossa** and draw a line along the medial edge of the **tendon of biceps femoris** to the inferior surface and posterior border of the **head of fibula**.
5. Continue the line inferior to the **head of fibula** and round the lateral aspect of the **neck of fibula** to the proximal part of the belly of **peroneus longus** (*Objective No 141*).
6. This line represents the course of the **common peroneal nerve**.

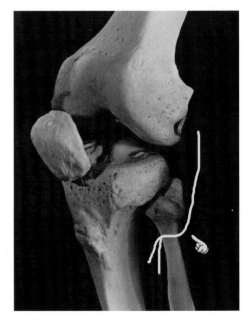

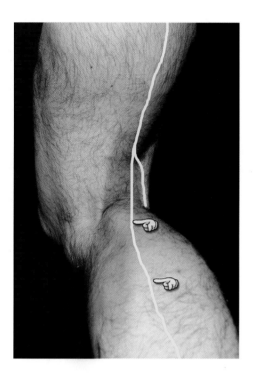

159. TIBIAL AND POSTERIOR TIBIAL NERVES

1. Ask the model to flex the **knee joint** to a right angle.
2. Identify and mark the boundaries of the **popliteal fossa**.
3. Identify and mark the **medial malleolus** and **medial tubercle of calcaneus**.
4. Draw a line connecting the **medial malleolus** to the **medial tubercle of calcaneus**.
5. Mark the midpoint of the line drawn in step 4.
6. Draw a line from a point just above the **apex of the popliteal fossa**, down the midline of the **popliteal fossa**.
7. Continue the line on the posterior surface of the **leg**, inclining towards the medial aspect of the **heel**, to join the midpoint of the line drawn in step 4.
8. The line drawn indicates the course of the **tibial nerve** and its continuation, the **posterior tibial nerve**.

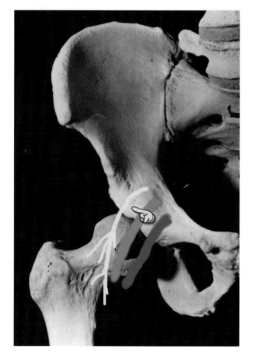

160. FEMORAL NERVE IN THE REGION OF THE HIP JOINT

1. Identify the pulse of the **femoral artery** and mark the position (*Objective No 153*).
2. Mark a point adjacent to the **femoral artery** on its lateral side.
3. At this point the **femoral nerve** enters **femoral triangle** of the **thigh** lying lateral to the **femoral artery** as it crosses the anterior aspect of the **hip joint**.

13

Bony Features of the Axial Skeleton (1)

161. SPINOUS PROCESSES C2–C6 OR C7

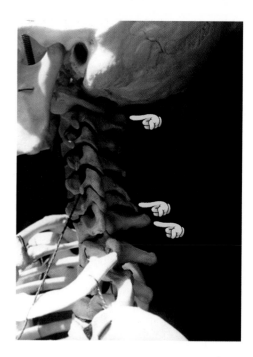

1. Place the model at rest, face down on a plinth with the **forehead** resting on the **dorsal surfaces** of the **hands**.
2. Place a pillow under the **ankles** to reduce muscle tone and ensure the model is comfortable.
3. Stand at the top (head) end of the plinth facing the model and complete the following steps:
   a. Identify by palpation the **external occipital protruberance**.
   b. Move the fingertips down the median **nuchal furrow** approximately 5 cm and identify the **spinous process of C2**.
   c. Palpate the **bifid spines of C3**, **C4** and **C5**, keeping one fingertip on the identified **spinous process** when palpating to identify the next structure.
   d. Identify the **spinous process of C6**, keeping fingertip contact, and ask the model to extend the **cervical spine**.
   e. The **spinous process of C6** appears to glide forwards while the **spinous process of C7** remains relatively fixed compared with **C6**.
   f. The **spinous process of C7** is the most prominent process.

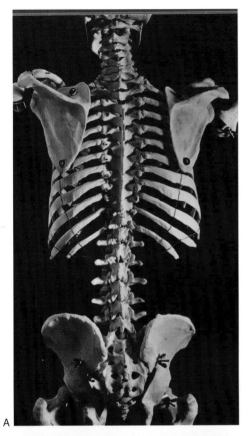

A

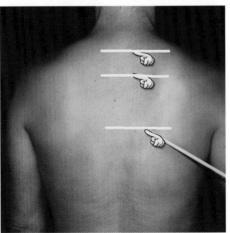

B

162. SPINOUS PROCESSES T1–T3, T7 OR T12

1. Ask the model to adduct and medially rotate the **glenohumeral joint**, fully flex the **elbow joint** and place one hand on the posterior surface of the **thorax** in the median plane.
2. Identify by palpation the **inferior angle of the scapula** and base of the **spine of scapula** by tracing the vertebral border upwards from the **inferior angle of the scapula** (*Objective No 1*).
3. Identify by palpation the position of the superior **angle of the scapula** which lies immediately superior to the **base of the spine of scapula**.
4. Ask the model to return to the anatomical position and mark the position of the **inferior** and **superior angles of the scapula**, the **vertebral border** and **base of the spine of scapula**.
5. Draw a vertical line from the **inferior angle of the scapula** downwards to cut the **iliac crest** and mark the midpoint of this line.
6. Draw a horizontal line from the midpoint of this vertical line to the median plane. This line meets the **spinous process** of the **12th thoracic vertebra**.
7. Draw a horizontal line from the **superior angle of the scapula** to the **median plane**. This line meets the **spinous process** of the **2nd thoracic vertebra**.
8. Draw a horizontal line from the **base of the spine of scapula** to the **median plane**. This line meets the **spinous process** of the **3rd thoracic vertebra**.
9. Draw a horizontal line from the **inferior angle of the scapula** to the **median plane**. This line meets the **spinous process** of the **7th thoracic vertebra**.
10. Ask the model to fully flex the **cervical and thoracic spines** and illuminate with side lighting.
11. Identify by palpation and mark the **spinous process** of the **7th cervical vertebra** (*Objective No 161*).
12. Palpate the **spinous process of C7** with the tip of the index finger and move down to the **spinous process of T1**, palpating with the tip of the middle finger.
13. Maintain palpation contact with the **spinous processes of C7 and T1** and palpate the **spinous process of T2**.
14. Repeat the palpation sequence, always keeping three fingertips in contact with the **spinous processes** to ensure recollection of previous structures identified in the sequence.

163. SPINOUS PROCESSES L2–L4 OR L5

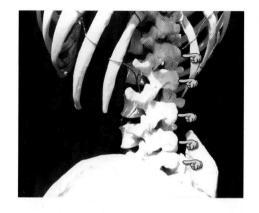

Part 1
1. Surface mark the outline of the right and left **iliac crests** (*Objective No 86*).
2. Surface mark the position of the summit of each **iliac crest** and draw a horizontal line connecting the summits across the **posterior aspect of the trunk**.
3. The horizontal line cuts the gap in the median plane between the **spinous processes** of the **3rd** and **4th lumbar vertebrae**.
4. Ask the model to take up the position of prone lying with comfortable support being placed to reduce **extensor muscle tone** in the **lumbar region**.
5. Palpate the ridge-like subcutaneous posterior **spinous processes** of the **lumbar vertebrae**, each process being approximately 10–15 mm in length with a gap between each of about 10 mm.
6. Place the thumb tips together against the lateral aspect of individual **lumbar spinous processes** and gently apply light pressure to identify the **interspinous gap** and edge of the ridge-like process.
7. The interspinous space is occupied by the **interspinous ligament** and the posterior edge of the ridge-like spinous process is covered by the **supraspinous ligament**.

Part 2
1. Identify and surface mark the outline of the **iliac crest** (*Objective No 86*).
2. Identify and surface mark the position of the **tubercles of the iliac crest** on both sides.
3. Draw a horizontal line connecting the **tubercles of the iliac crests**.
4. Palpate and mark the point where the horizontal line crosses the median plane on the posterior aspect of the **trunk**.
5. At the point marked in step 4, the line cuts the upper border of the **spinous process** of the **5th lumbar vertebra**.
6. Place the model in prone lying with comfortable support to reduce **extensor muscle** tone.
7. Palpate the distinct horizontal subcutaneous bony upper border of the **1st sacral vertebra** in the median plane.
8. Palpate upwards in the midline and identify the **spinous process** of the **5th lumbar vertebra**, which lies approximately 12 mm superior to the **1st sacral vertebra**.

164. BODY OF RIBS 1–7, 11 AND 12

This objective is in four parts:
- 1st rib
- 2nd rib
- 3rd to 7th ribs
- 11th and 12th ribs.

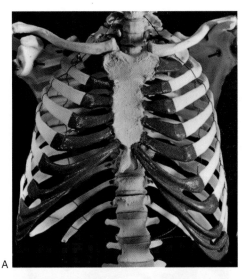

A

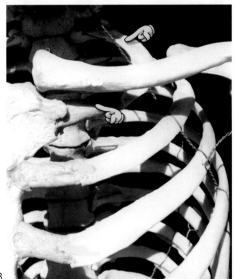

B

1st rib

1. Place the palm of the hand on the **shoulder** with the palmar surface of the fingers on the posterior aspect of the **upper fibres of trapezius** and the thumb resting on the superior border of the **clavicle** with the thumb tip in the **supraclavicular fossa** lateral to the **sternocleidomastoid** (*Objective No 174*).
2. Gently press the thumb tip downwards and in a posterior direction until springy resistance is encountered.
3. This resistance is due to the body of the **1st rib**. Mark this position with a pen.
4. The pulse of the **subclavian artery** may be counted at this point as the artery crosses over the body of the **1st rib** (*Objective No 186*).

2nd rib

1. Palpate the **sternal angle** and surface mark (*Objective No 166*).
2. Mark the position of the median plane where it cuts the **sternal angle**.
3. Palpate in a lateral direction from the median plane along the **sternal angle** to the **2nd costal cartilage** where it joins the lateral border of the **sternum**.
4. Continue in a lateral direction along the **costal cartilage** of the **2nd rib** to the **mid-clavicular line**.
5. The body of the **2nd rib** can be palpated from its junction with the **2nd costal cartilage** to the **mid-clavicular line** and identified as a spring-like resistance under the light pressure of the palpating fingertip.
6. The **1st intercostal space** lies between the **1st** and **2nd costal cartilages** and bodies of the **ribs**.

3rd to 7th ribs

1. Identify and surface mark the outline of the **clavicle**.
2. Draw a vertical line at the midpoint of the **clavicle** on the anterior surface of the **thorax** representing the **mid-clavicular line**.
3. Identify and surface mark the **sternal angle** then trace the **2nd costal cartilage** to the body of the **2nd rib**.
4. Identify and surface mark the position of the body of the **2nd rib** in the **mid-clavicular line**.
5. Mark the position of the **1st intercostal space** in the **mid-clavicular line** superior to the body of the **2nd rib** and inferior to the body of the **1st rib**.
6. Mark the position of the **2nd intercostal space** in the **mid-clavicular line** superior to the body of the **3rd rib** and inferior to the body of the **2nd rib** in the **mid-clavicular line**.
7. Identify and surface mark the body of the **3rd rib** in the **mid-clavicular line**.
8. Identify and surface mark the position of the **4th intercostal space** inferior to the body of the **3rd rib** in the **mid-clavicular line**.
9. Draw a vertical line on the anterior aspect of the **thorax** representing the lateral vertical plane drawn at the midpoint between the median plane and the **acromion process of scapula** (*Objective No 4*).

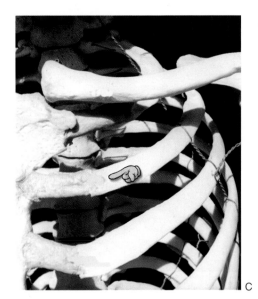

C

10. From the **4th intercostal space** move in a lateral direction to the lateral vertical plane and identify the body of the **5th rib** and surface mark.
11. From the body of the **5th rib** surface marked in the lateral vertical plane, palpate the **5th intercostal space** and surface mark the body of the **6th rib**.
12. Palpate the **6th intercostal space** inferior to the body of the **6th rib** in the **lateral vertical plane**.
13. Mark the position of the body of the **7th rib** in the lateral vertical plane and move the palpating fingertip in a medial direction crossing the **mid-clavicular line** towards the **costal margin**.
14. Trace the **costal cartilage** of the **7th rib** to where the **costal cartilage** meets the inferior and lateral margins of the body of the **sternum** adjacent to the **xiphisternal synchondrosis**.
15. The **xiphisternal synchondrosis** is a fused **secondary cartilaginous joint** formed in the midline between the body of the **sternum** and the **xiphoid process**. This joint can be identified by palpation as a raised horizontal ridge approximately 15 mm long just medial and inferior to the junction of the **7th costal cartilage** of the **7th rib** with the body of the **sternum**.

11th and 12th ribs
1. Place the model in prone lying with comfortable supports to reduce muscle tone.
2. Place the nail surfaces of both thumbs together and lightly rest on the median plane in the **lumbar furrow**.
3. Place the palmar surfaces of both hands lightly on the **lumbar** area, fingers together, with the medial surfaces of the little fingers resting on the posterior one-third of the **iliac crests** (*Objective No 86*).
4. Firm, gentle, gradual and deep palpation pressure upwards and in a medial direction on the **abdominal muscles** with the lateral surface of the index fingers is met by a firm spring-like resistance.
5. This resistance, encountered on palpation from the lateral margin of the **sacrospinalis muscles**, is the body of the **12th rib** and can be identified forwards to, and occasionally beyond, the **mid-axillary line** to the **costal cartilage** tip of the **12th rib**, which is free and unattached.
6. The **11th intercostal space** can be identified as a gap at the lateral margin of **sacrospinalis** lying superior to the body of the **12th rib** and inferior to the inferior border of the **11th rib** which can be identified above.
7. Palpate gently upwards with the index finger to identify the body of the **11th rib** and trace the bony contour forwards towards and occasionally beyond the **mid-axillary line** to its anterior extremity, terminating in **costal cartilage**, which is free and unattached.

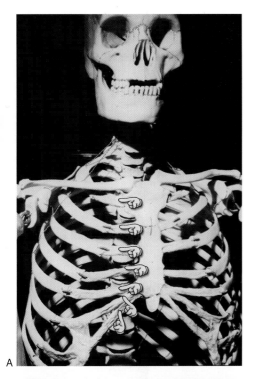

A

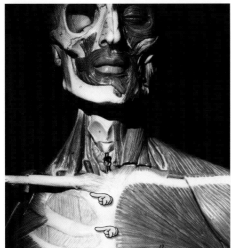

B

165. COSTAL CARTILAGES 1–6 OR 7

1. Identify and surface mark the medial extremity of the **clavicle** (*Objective No 2*).
2. Palpate immediately below the inferior border of the medial extremity of the **clavicle**.
3. Identify and mark the structure which articulates with the **manubrium of the sternum** and is the **1st costal cartilage**.
4. Place the tip of the ring finger on the **1st costal cartilage** and the middle finger on the **1st intercostal space** immediately below.
5. Maintaining the fingers in this position, place the tip of the index finger on the **2nd costal cartilage** which articulates with the **sternum** at the **sternal angle** (*Objective No 166*).
6. Replace the tip of the index finger on the **2nd costal cartilage** with the ring finger and identify the **2nd intercostal space** lying immediately inferior with the middle finger.
7. Place the tip of the index finger on the **3rd costal cartilage** lying below and mark the position of the **three costal cartilages**.
8. Commence palpation again and place tip of the index finger on the **3rd intercostal space** and surface mark.
9. Repeat the process, always keeping one finger in contact with the previous structure. The **4th costal cartilage** can be identified and marked below the **3rd intercostal space**.
10. Palpate the costal margin and identify the **7th (last) costal cartilage** articulating directly with the **sternum** and surface mark.
11. The **5th** and **6th costal cartilages** articulate directly with the body of the **sternum** but as they near the lateral border of the **sternum** the **intercostal spaces** become indistinct.
12. Change the procedure and draw a vertical line to represent the **mid-clavicular line**.
13. Identify the **sternal angle** and the **2nd costal cartilage**. Move in a lateral direction towards the **mid-clavicular line** along the body of the **2nd rib**.
14. Palpate and surface mark the body of the **2nd**, **3rd** and **4th ribs** and related **intercostal spaces** until the body of the **5th rib** is palpated and surface marked.
15. Palpate the body of the **5th rib** and move towards the median plane until the **costal cartilage** and lateral margin of the **sternum** are reached. Surface mark.
16. Move back to the **mid-clavicular line**; identify the **5th intercostal space** and, below, the body of the **6th rib** and surface mark.
17. Palpate the body of the **6th rib** and move in a medial direction towards the median plane until the **costal cartilage** and lateral margin of the **sternum** are reached. Surface mark.

166. STERNAL ANGLE

1. Identify the **jugular notch** and surface mark.
2. Draw a line to represent the median plane from the **jugular notch** to the **xiphisternal synchondrosis** (*Objective No 167*).
3. Palpate the **jugular notch** and move the fingertip down the median plane for a distance of approximately 5 cm until a horizontal raised ridge is encountered lying across the median plane and surface mark.
4. This raised ridge is a **secondary cartilaginous joint** formed between the **manubrium and body** (gladiolus) of the **sternum**.
5. The **2nd costal cartilage** articulates with the **sternum** at the **sternal angle**.

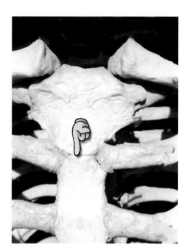

167. XIPHISTERNAL SYNCHONDROSIS

1. Ask the model to take up a position of supine lying on a plinth with comfortable support for the **knees** and **cervical spine** to reduce muscle tone in the **abdominal muscles**.
2. Draw a vertical line from the **jugular notch** to the **umbilicus** to represent the median plane.
3. Gently palpate the costal margin towards the median plane and identify the **9th costal cartilage** where it is cut by the lateral margin of **rectus abdominis** (*Objective No 180*).
4. Continue to palpate upwards and towards the median plane palpating the **8th** and **7th costal cartilage**.
5. Mark the position where the **7th costal cartilage** meets the **sternum**.
6. Palpate towards the median plane and slightly change the direction of palpation, moving upwards and medially to identify a horizontal ridge approximately 1.5 cm long lying across the median plane, and surface mark.
7. This short horizontal ridge marks the position of the **secondary cartilaginous joint** which is the **xiphisternal synchondrosis**.

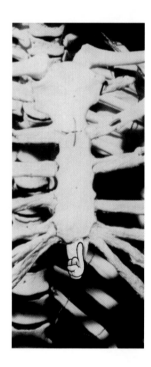

14

Bony Features of the Axial Skeleton (2)

168. MASTOID PROCESS

1. Ask the model to demonstrate the action of the **sternocleidomastoid muscle**.
2. Palpate the **muscle** from its **clavicular attachment** upwards to its attachment on the **temporal bone** behind the **lobule** and lower part of the **concha of the auricle**.
3. Palpate behind the **concha of the auricle** and identify a prominent subcutaneous bony mass, which is the **mastoid process** of the **temporal bone**, and surface mark.

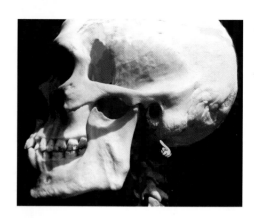

169. ANGLE OF THE MANDIBLE

1. Palpate and mark the point of the **chin** in the midline.
2. Palpate in a posterior direction along the inferior border of the **body of the mandible**, crossing an indentation where the pulse of the **facial artery** can be identified.
3. Continue palpating in a posterior direction along the inferior border to a point where the bone changes direction upwards and starts to form the **ramus of the mandible**.
4. The prominent subcutaneous angle palpated at this point where there is a change of direction is the **angle of the mandible**.

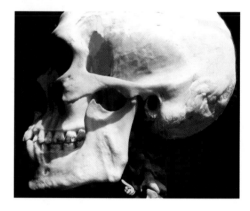

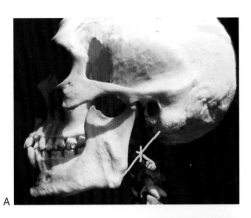

A

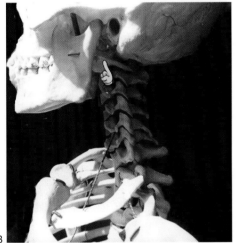

B

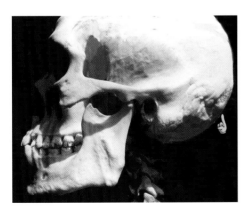

170. TRANSVERSE PROCESS OF C1

Note: Caution is to be observed and gentle palpation is required.

1. Identify and mark the **angle of the mandible** (*Objective No 169*).
2. Identify and mark the tip of the **mastoid process** (*Objective No 168*).
3. Draw a line connecting the points in steps 1 and 2 passing behind the **ear**.
4. Mark a point midway between the tip of the **mastoid process** and the **angle of the mandible**.
5. Gently and with a light touch, palpate into the substance of the **parotid gland**.
6. Palpate gently until resistance is encountered.
7. The resistance to the palpating finger is produced by the tip of the **lateral process of the 1st cervical vertebra**.

171. EXTERNAL OCCIPITAL PROTRUBERANCE

1. Ask the model to assume a comfortable and supported position in prone lying with the forehead resting on the **dorsum of the hands**.
2. Ask the model to extend the **cervical spine**; identify and mark the position of the **nuchal furrow**.
3. Palpate the **nuchal furrow** from below upwards to the **occipital bone**.
4. Palpate the upper area of the **nuchal furrow** in the midline and identify a prominent and elevated bony feature on the **occipital bone**.
5. This raised, subcutaneous bony feature is the **external occipital protruberance** and is easily identified when palpated from below.
6. The highest point on this feature in the midline is known as the **inion**.

172. ZYGOMATIC ARCH

1. Identify the **external auditory meatus of the ear**.
2. Palpate the **tragus of the ear**.
3. Identify and mark the **temporomandibular joint line** 1 cm anterior to the **tragus of the ear**.
4. Draw a horizontal line from the **temporomandibular joint** to the bony prominence of the **zygomatic bone** (*Objective No 173*).
5. Palpate with the fingertips along this line, identify and mark a prominent bony ridge, the **zygomatic arch**.
6. On clenching the **teeth** the **temporalis muscle** can be identified **superior** to the zygomatic arch.
7. On clenching the **teeth** the **masseter muscle** can be identified **inferior** to the zygomatic arch.

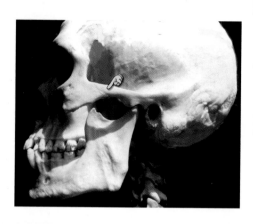

173. ZYGOMA

1. Place the palpating fingertip on and mark the bony subcutaneous prominence of the **cheek** placed 1.5 cm below and lateral to the **infraorbital margin**.
2. Palpate and surface mark the lateral surface of the **zygomatic bone**, tracing it superiorly into the frontal process, posteriorly into the **zygomatic arch** and anteriorly into the **zygomatic process of the maxilla**.

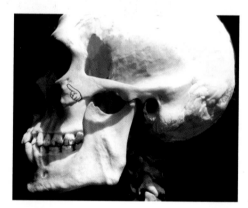

15

Muscles of the Neck, Trunk and Abdomen

174. STERNOCLEIDOMASTOID

1. Surface mark the **mastoid process** (*Objective No 168*), **clavicle** (*Objective No 2*) and **manubrium of sternum** (*Objective No 166*).
2. Ask the model to flex the **cervical spine** to one side and the rotate the **cervical spine** to the opposite side against maximal resistance.
3. Palpate the muscle fibres passing from the **mastoid process** and **occipital bone** to their inferior attachments on the medial extremity of the **clavicle** and **manubrium of sternum**.
4. Observe how the borders of **sternocleidomastoid** form a boundary of the **posterior** and **anterior triangles of the neck**.

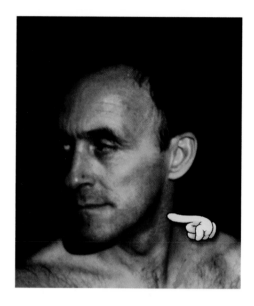

175. SCALENE

1. Identify the boundaries of the **posterior triangle of the neck** (*Objective No 201*).
2. Ask the model to flex the **cervical spine** to one side and elevate the **shoulder** against maximal resistance.
3. Palpate the contracting muscle fibres as they pass to their separate attachments on the **1st** and **2nd ribs** between the anterior border of the **upper fibres of trapezius** and the posterior border of **sternocleidomastoid**.

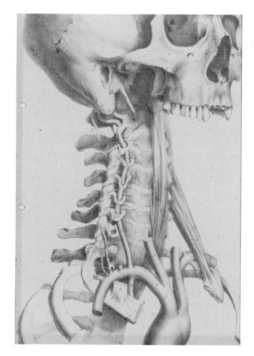

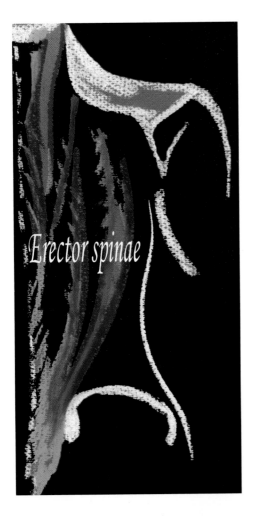

176. ERECTOR SPINAE

1. Ask the model to take up the position of prone lying.
2. Ask the model to fully extend the joints of the **vertebral column** against gravity.
3. Observe and palpate the parallel contours of **erector spinae** formed in the **lumbar** and **lower thoracic** sections as two distinct vertical columns on each side of the **vertebral column**.
4. Side flexion and rotation of the **vertebral column** to one side against maximal resistance will bring **erector spinae** into action.

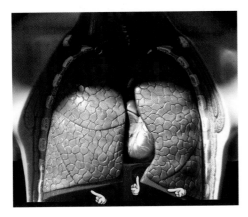

177. DIAPHRAGM

1. Ask the model take up a position of supine lying with **head** and **shoulders** raised, **knees** slightly flexed and comfortably supported to reduce **abdominal muscle** tone.
2. Place a small pillow to support and maintain the normal **lumbar curve**.
3. Place light manual resistance against the **lower abdominal wall** on each side of the midline.
4. Ask the model to inspire and, maintaining the **lumbar spine** position, to gently push out against the resistance placed against the lower abdominal wall as inspiration takes place.

178. EXTERNAL ABDOMINAL OBLIQUE

1. Ask the model to take up a position of supine lying with **legs** astride.
2. Ask the model to touch the **left foot** with the **right hand** to demonstrate the action of the **right external abdominal oblique** working with the **left internal abdominal oblique**.
3. Palpate the **external abdominal oblique** at its attachments to the **lower eight ribs** where it interdigitates with the **fibres of serratus anterior**.
4. Palpate obliquely downwards towards the **rectus abdominis** where it assists in forming the **sheath of rectus**.

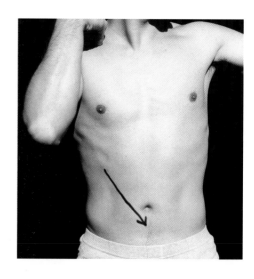

179. INTERNAL ABDOMINAL OBLIQUE

1. Ask the model to take up a position of supine lying with **legs** astride.
2. Ask the model to touch the **left foot** with the **right hand** to demonstrate the action of the **left internal abdominal oblique** working with the **right external abdominal oblique**.
3. The **internal abdominal oblique** is situated below the **external abdominal oblique** and fibres pass from the **iliac crest, inguinal ligament and fascia** towards the **pubis, rectus abdominis** (where it participates in forming the sheath of **rectus abdominis**) and the **costal cartilages** of the **9th, 10th, 11th** and **12th ribs**.

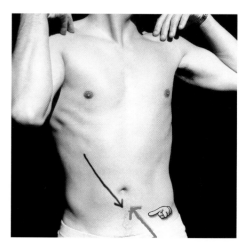

180. RECTUS ABDOMINIS

1. Ask the model to take up a position of supine lying.
2. Ask the model to flex the **thoracic** and **lumbar** sections of the **vertebral column** against gravity.
3. **Rectus abdominis** can be palpated on each side of the midline from the **xiphoid process** and **costal cartilages** of the **5th, 6th** and **7th ribs** to its attachment on the **crest of pubis**.

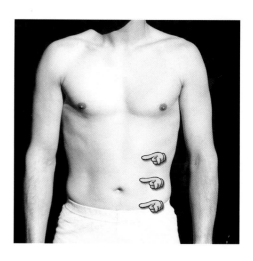

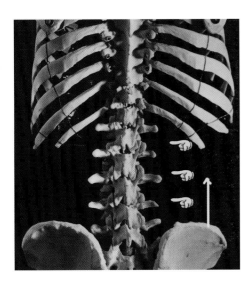

181. QUADRATUS LUMBORUM

1. Ask the model to weight bear on one **foot**.
2. **Quadratus lumborum** acts on the non-weight-bearing side to maintain the **pelvis** level and the **anterior superior iliac spines** in the same horizontal plane.
3. **Quadratus lumborum** acts with **gluteus medius** of the opposite side to maintain the **pelvis** level during walking and similar activities of locomotion.
4. **Quadratus lumborum** can be palpated immediately lateral to the **erector spinae** as fibres pass downwards from the **12th rib**, and transverse processes of the **upper four lumbar vertebrae** to its inferior attachments on the **iliac crest** and **iliolumbar ligament**.

16

Arteries of the Head and Neck

182. COMMON CAROTID

Note: Do not compress the common carotid artery against the prominent anterior tubercle of the transverse process of the 6th cervical vertebra.

Note: The common carotid arteries are situated on each side of the trachea (*Objective No 199*).

1. Draw a vertical line to represent the median plane from the **jugular notch** to the **mentis**.
2. Ask the model to rotate the **cervical spine** and surface mark the **anterior border of sternocleidomastoid** (*Objective No 174*).
3. Surface mark the **articular process**, **ramus** and **body of the mandible**.
4. Surface mark the **sternoclavicular joint** (*Objective No 21*).
5. Palpate and mark the upper border of the **thyroid cartilage**.
6. Draw a line from the **sternoclavicular joint** to the depression between the **angle of the mandible** and the **mastoid process**.
7. Palpate the upper lateral border of the **thyroid cartilage**.
8. The **common carotid artery** corresponds to the line in step 6. At the level of the upper border of the **thyroid cartilage**, the **common carotid** usually divides into the **internal** and **external** carotid arteries.

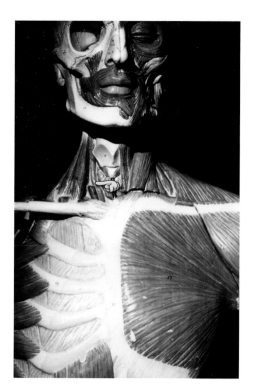

183. EXTERNAL CAROTID

1. Identify the superior border of the **thyroid cartilage** in the **anterior triangle of the neck**.
2. Identify and mark the position of the **head** and **neck of mandible**.
3. Draw a line from the upper border of the thyroid cartilage to the **neck of mandible**.
4. This line corresponds to the course of the **external carotid artery** in the **anterior triangle of the neck**.

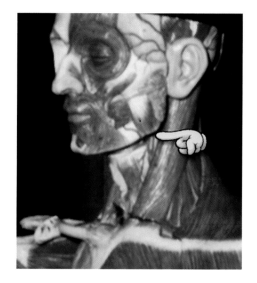

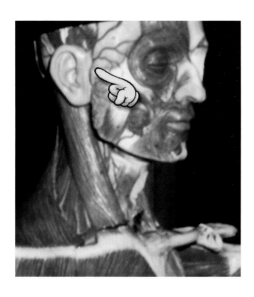

184. SUPERFICIAL TEMPORAL

1. Identify and surface mark the position of the **neck of mandible** (*Objective No 183*).
2. Identify and mark the **temporomandibular joint** line.
3. Identify the pulse of the **superficial temporal artery** as it passes over the root of the **zygomatic process** anterior to the **temporomandibular joint**.

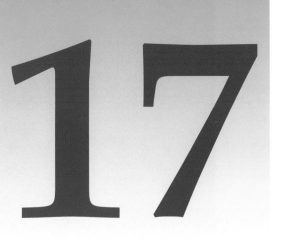

Organs (1)

185. BRACHIAL PLEXUS

1. Ask the model to rotate the **cervical spine** to the right through 70° and side flex to the left against slight resistance to demonstrate the action of the **left sternocleidomastoid** (*Objective No 174*).
2. Mark the posterior border of the **sternocleidomastoid, superior border of the shaft of clavicle** (*Objective No 2*) and **anterior border of the upper fibres of trapezius** (*Objective No 29*).
3. Note the position and borders of the above structures which form the **posterior triangle of the neck**.
4. Identify and mark the midpoint of the **posterior border of sternocleidomastoid**.
5. Identify and mark the midpoint of the **shaft of clavicle**.
6. Draw a line between the marked points in steps 4 and 5.
7. The trunks of the **brachial plexus** pass downwards and in a lateral direction within the **supraclavicular area** (as marked out in steps 4, 5 and 6) of the **posterior triangle of the neck**.
8. The trunks of the **brachial plexus** pass between the **clavicle** and **1st rib** into the **axilla** and form three cords.

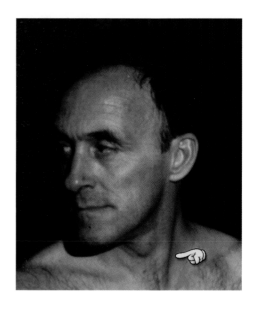

186. SUBCLAVIAN ARTERY

1. Identify the **jugular notch** of the **manubrium** in the **median plane**.
2. Move the palpating fingertip in a lateral direction and identify the line of the **sternoclavicular joint** (*Objective No 21*).
3. Draw a curved line from the **sternoclavicular joint** to the midpoint of the **shaft of clavicle**.
4. Ensure that the convexity of the line is upwards into the **supraclavicular fossa** to a point approximately 2 cm above the midpoint of the **shaft of clavicle**.
5. Draw the line curving downwards to terminate at the lateral border of the body of the **1st rib** (*Objective No 164*).

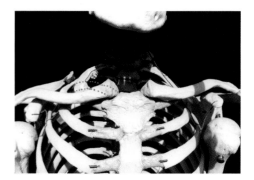

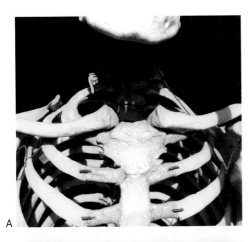

A

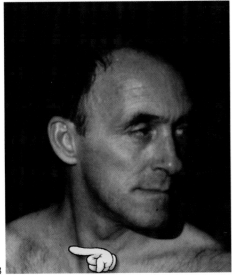

B

187. UPPER LOBE APICAL SEGMENT

1. Identify and mark the **superior border of clavicle** (*Objective No 2*).
2. Ask the model to depress both **clavicles** to the same horizontal plane.
3. Demonstrate and mark the **clavicular attachment** of the **sternocleidomastoid muscle** (*Objective No 174*).
4. Mark a point in the **supraclavicular fossa** 3 cm superior to the **medial one-third of the clavicle** and **clavicular attachment of sternocleidomastoid**.
5. Draw a line from the marked point in step 4 to cut the **sternoclavicular joint** (*Objective No 21*).
6. Draw a line from the marked point in step 4 to the outer border of the body of the **1st rib** (*Objective No 164*).
7. These two lines represent the projected borders of the apex of the upper lobes of the **right and left lungs**.

188. LOWER LOBE APICAL SEGMENT

1. Identify and mark the tip of the **spinous process** of the **2nd thoracic vertebra**.
2. Draw a curved line to represent the upper one-third of the **oblique fissure** of the **lung** (*Objective No 189*).
3. Draw a vertical line 2.5 cm lateral to the median plane starting on a level with the **spinous process** of the **2nd thoracic vertebra** to point on a level with the **spinous process** of the **5th thoracic vertebra**.
4. This triangular area represents the apex of the **lower lobe of the lung** lying immediately inferior and lateral to the **spinous process** of the **2nd thoracic vertebra** below the **oblique fissure**.

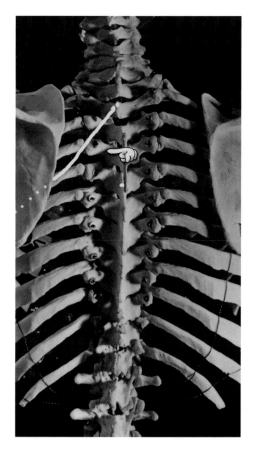

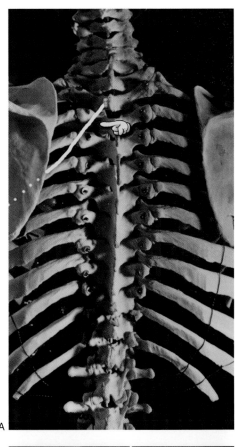

A

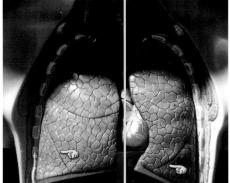

B

189. OBLIQUE FISSURE OF THE LUNG

1. Identify and mark the tip of the **spinous process** of the **2nd thoracic vertebra** (*Objective No 162*).
2. Identify and mark a point 2 cm lateral to the tip of the **spinous process** of the **2nd thoracic vertebra**.
3. Identify and mark the position of the **6th sternocostal junction**.
4. Ask the model to fully elevate the upper limb so that the **scapula** is rotated.
5. Draw a curving line round the **thoracic wall** from point 2 to point 3.
6. This line passes downwards and outwards parallel to the **vertebral border of scapula** to the **inferior angle of scapula**, crosses the body of the **5th rib** in the **mid-axillary line** and terminates at the **6th sternocostal junction** at the **inferior border of the lung** 7.5 cm from the median plane.

190. TRANSVERSE/HORIZONTAL FISSURE OF RIGHT LUNG

1. Ask the model to fully elevate the right **upper limb**.
2. Draw a vertical line to represent the **right mid-axillary line**.
3. Identify and mark the body of the **5th rib** at the point where it is cut by the **mid-axillary line**.
4. Identify and mark the lower border of the body of the **4th rib** and the **4th costal cartilage**.
5. Draw a line passing from the marked point in step 3 transversely along the lower border of the **4th rib** to the **4th costal cartilage** where it terminates at the anterior margin to represent the **transverse/horizontal fissure of right lung**.

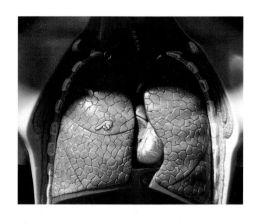

191. OUTLINE OF THE HEART – APEX BEAT OF THE HEART

1. Palpate and mark the lower border of the **second left costal cartilage** 2 cm from the **left border** of the **sternum** (*Objective No 166*).
2. Palpate and mark the upper border of the **3rd right costal cartilage** 1.5 cm from the **right border of the sternum**.
3. Palpate and mark the lower border of the **6th right costal cartilage** 2 cm from the **right border of the sternum**.
4. Palpate and mark the position of the **5th left intercostal space** 10 cm from the median plane.
5. Observe, listen to and mark the **apex beat of the heart** in the **5th left interspace** 9 cm from the median plane.
6. Connect the marked points in steps 1 and 2 with a straight line.
7. Connect the marked points in steps 2 and 3 by a curved line. Greatest point of curvature is 3.5 cm in the **4th interspace**.
8. Connect the marked points in steps 3 and 4 with a line presenting a slight downward convexity passing just superior to the **xiphisternal synchondrosis** (*Objective No 167*).
9. Connect the marked points in steps 1 and 4 with a line presenting a convexity to the left.

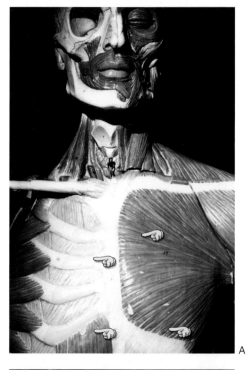

A

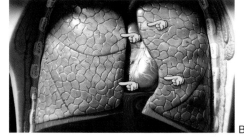

B

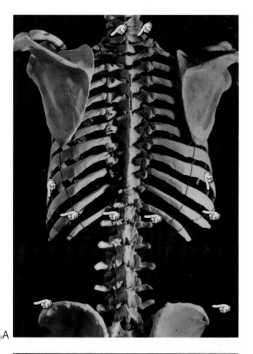

A

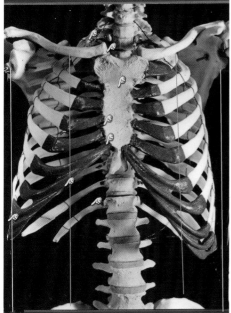

B

192. PARIETAL PLEURA LIMITS OF THE LUNGS

Note: The left and right parietal pleura are different.

Right parietal pleura

1. Palpate and mark the tip of the **7th cervical spinous process** (*Objective No 161*).
2. Mark a point 2.5 cm lateral to the tip of the **7th cervical spinous process**.
3. Mark a point 3.5 cm above the junction of the medial one-third and mid-third of the **shaft of clavicle. Note the clavicular attachment of sternocleidomastoid.**
4. From the marked point in step 3 draw a line to the **sternoclavicular joint**.
5. Identify the **jugular notch** and palpate downwards on the **manubrium of the sternum** for about 5 cm to the **sternal angle** which is marked by a horizontal ridge in the median plane.
6. Draw a line from the **sternoclavicular joint** to a point where the **sternal angle** is cut by the median plane.
7. Identify the **2nd costal cartilage** where it articulates with the **sternal angle** and count down to the **6th costal cartilage** and mark.
8. Identify and mark the midpoint of the **shaft of clavicle**.
9. Draw a vertical line from the marked point in step 8 on the **thorax** to cut the body of the **8th rib** and mark this point.
10. Identify the **axillary space** and surface mark the **mid-axillary line** to where it cuts the **iliac crest**.
11. Count down and mark the **10th intercostal space**.
12. Draw a vertical line from the **inferior angle of scapula** downwards to where it cuts the **11th intercostal space**.
13. Mark a point 2 cm lateral to the tip of the **12th thoracic spinous process**.
14. Connect all the above points with a final line from No 13 to No 2.

Note: The inferior border of the pleura lies below the body of the 12th rib.

Left parietal pleura

1. Ask the model to depress both **shoulders** to bring the **clavicles** to a horizontal plane.
2. Mark the **clavicular attachment** of the left **sternocleidomastoid muscle**.
3. Mark a point 3.5 cm superior to the **clavicular attachment** of the left **sternocleidomastoid muscle**.
4. Surface mark the left **sternoclavicular joint** line.
5. Draw the line of the median plane where it cuts the **sternal angle**.
6. Surface mark the left **4th costosternal junction**.
7. Draw a line to represent the **left lateral vertical plane** on the anterior surface of the **thorax**.
8. Surface mark the positions of the **left 5th**, **6th** and **7th costal cartilages**.
9. Draw a vertical line to indicate the position of the left

mid-axillary line on the surface of the **thorax**.

10. Draw a vertical line cutting the inferior angle of the left **scapula** on the surface of the **thorax**.
11. Identify and surface mark the position of the body of the **12th rib**.
12. Identify and mark the left lateral border of the **erector spinae muscles**.
13. Draw a line from the marked point in step 3 downwards and medially to cut the **sternoclavicular joint**.
14. Continue the line from the marked point in step 4 to that in step 5 and mark where the **median plane** cuts the **sternal angle**.
15. The lines of the **left parietal pleura** and **right parietal pleura** converge slightly to the left of the median plane.
16. Continue the line vertically downwards to the **4th costal cartilage** surface marked in step 6.
17. Continue the line downwards and obliquely outwards crossing the **5th**, **6th** and **7th costal cartilages** as surface marked in step 8.
18. Draw the line to meet the left lateral vertical line at the **8th costal cartilage**.
19. Continue the line to the **mid-axillary line** where it cuts the body of the **10th rib**.
20. Draw the line from the marked point in step 7 to the body of the **12th rib** at the lateral border of the **erector spinae muscles**.
21. Finally draw a vertical line upwards from the marked point in step 8 to meet the original starting point 3.5 cm above the **clavicular attachment** of the left **sternocleidomastoid muscle** on a level with the **spinous process of C7**, 2.5 cm from the median plane.

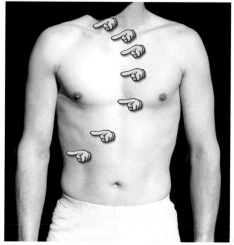

B

18

Organs (2)

193. SPLEEN

1. Ask the model to fully abduct the **left upper limb**.
2. Draw a vertical line to represent the **left mid-axillary line**.
3. Identify by palpation and mark the position of the body of the **left 10th rib**.
4. Mark the position of the upper border of the body of the **left 11th rib**.
5. Mark the position of the lower border of the body of the **left 9th rib**.
6. Mark the long axis of the **spleen** which is in line with the body of the **10th rib**.
7. Mark the upper border of the **spleen** which extends to the upper border of the body of the **9th rib**.
8. Mark the lower border of the **spleen** which extends to the inferior border of the body of the **11th rib**.
9. Mark the anterior margin of the **spleen** which extends to the **left mid-axillary line**.
10. Mark the posterior margin of the **spleen** which lies approximately 5 cm lateral to the **spinous process of the 10th thoracic vertebra**.
11. Connect the borders and margins to form an oval shape 7.5 cm in width and 12.5 cm in length.

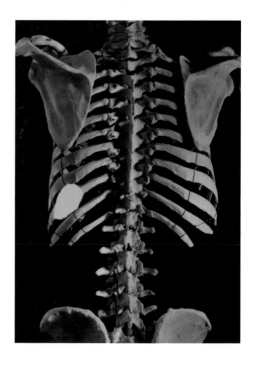

194. LIVER

1. Draw a line to represent the superior border from a point in the **left 5th intercostal space** 9 cm from the median plane cutting the **right 6th sternocostal junction** to the upper border of the **right 5th costal cartilage** in the lateral vertical plane and on to the body of the **6th rib in the mid-axillary line**.
2. Draw a line to represent the anterior border from a point in the **left 5th intercostal space** 9 cm from the median plane across the tip of the **left 8th costal cartilage** to the tip of the **right 9th costal cartilage**, and continue the line along the lower limit of the costal margin to the **mid-axillary line**.
3. Draw two vertical lines to represent the **right** and **left mid-axillary lines**.
4. Connect steps 1, 2 and 3.

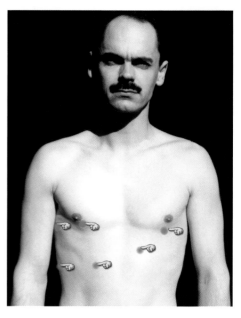

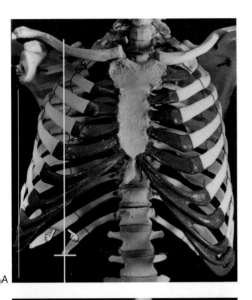

A

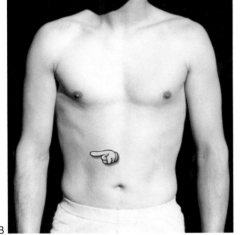

B

195. GALL BLADDER

1. Ask the model to demonstrate the action of the **rectus abdominis muscle** (*Objective No 180*).
2. Surface mark the position of the **right lateral margin of rectus abdominis**.
3. Identify by palpation and mark the tips of the **right 9th and 10th costal cartilages**.
4. Mark the position where the tip of the **right 9th costal cartilage** is cut by the **lateral margin of the rectus abdominis muscle**.
5. The fundus of the gall bladder projects from under the **anterior border of the liver** in the angle between the tips of the **right 9th and 10th costal cartilages** and the **lateral margin of rectus abdominis**.

196. KIDNEYS

1. Draw a vertical line to represent the posterior median plane.
2. Identify and mark the tip of the **spinous process** of the **11th thoracic vertebra**.
3. Identify and mark the posterior edge of the **spinous process** of the **3rd lumbar vertebra** (*Objective No 163*).
4. Draw two horizontal lines, one through the structure identified in step 2, and one through the structure identified in step 3.
5. Draw a vertical line on each side 3 cm from the median plane to levels identified in step 4.
6. Draw a vertical line on each side 9 cm from the median plane to levels identified in step 4.
7. Within the quadrilateral drawn on each side of the median plane the **right kidney** is placed slightly lower than the **left kidney** because of the mass of the liver above.
8. The long axis of each **kidney** is slightly inclined with the upper pole towards the median plane.

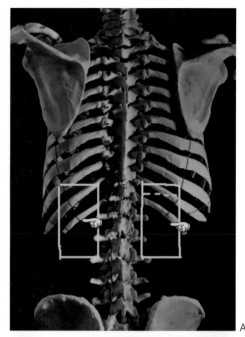

A

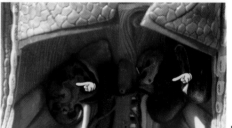

B

197. THYROID GLAND

1. Identify and mark the arch of the **cricoid cartilage** in the median plane.
2. Draw a 1.5 cm horizontal line, 1 cm inferior to the arch of the **cricoid cartilage** in the median plane.
3. Draw a 1.5 cm horizontal line, 2 cm inferior to the arch of the **cricoid cartilage** in the median plane.
4. The upper pole of the lateral lobe lies on a level with the **laryngeal prominence** adjacent to the anterior border of the **sternocleidomastoid muscle** (*Objective No 174*).
5. The lower pole of the lateral lobe projects downwards from the **isthmus** for approximately 1.5 cm.

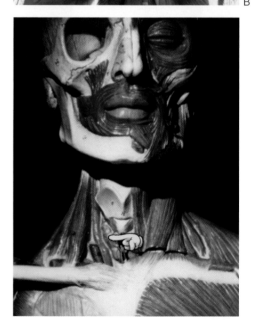

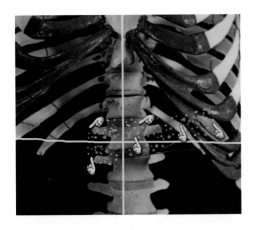

198. PANCREAS

1. Identify the position of the **spleen** (*Objective No 193*).
2. Draw a vertical line to represent the median plane.
3. Draw a horizontal line midway between the **jugular notch** and the **symphysis pubis** to represent the **transpyloric plane** cutting the body of the **1st lumbar vertebra**.
4. Draw two parallel lines 3 cm apart from the **hilum of the spleen** downwards and medially for 12 cm towards the **transpyloric plane** to cross the median plane (**these lines represent the tail, body and part of the neck of pancreas**).
5. **The head, uncinate process** and part of the **neck of pancreas** are positioned approximately 2.5 cm to the right of the median plane, on and slightly below the **transpyloric plane**.

199. TRACHEA

1. Identify and mark the arch of the **cricoid cartilage** in the median plane.
2. Draw two parallel lines 2 cm apart commencing immediately inferior to the **cricoid cartilage**.
3. Continue these two lines downwards, inclining very slightly to the right.
4. Terminate the two lines at the level of the **sternal angle** (*Objective No 166*) where the **trachea bifurcates** (**the carina**).

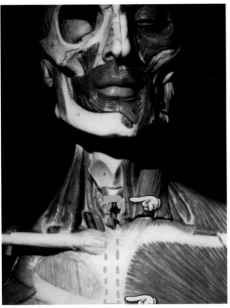

A

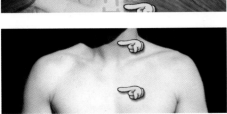

B

200. PYLORIC AND CARDIAC OPENINGS

1. Identify and mark the **xiphisternal synchondrosis**.
2. Draw a vertical line to represent the median plane.
3. Identify and mark the **left 7th costal cartilage**.
4. Mark a point 2.5 cm to the left of the median plane on the **7th costal cartilage** and about 1.5 cm to the left of the **xiphisternal synchondrosis**.
5. Draw two short parallel lines 2 cm apart downwards and to the left to represent the **cardiac opening**.
6. Draw a horizontal line to represent the **transpyloric plane** cutting the body of the **1st lumbar vertebra**.
7. Mark a point 1.2 cm to the right of the median plane on the **transpyloric plane**.
8. Draw two short parallel lines 2 cm apart directed upwards and to the right to represent the **pyloric opening**.

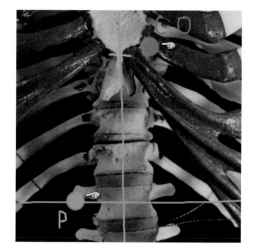

19

Anatomical Spaces

201. POSTERIOR TRIANGLE OF THE NECK

1. Draw a line to represent the anterior boundary along the posterior border of **sternocleidomastoid muscle**.
2. Draw a line to represent the posterior boundary along the anterior border of the **upper fibres of trapezius**.
3. Draw a line to represent the base of the **posterior triangle of the neck** along the **superior border of the middle third of the shaft of clavicle**.
4. Identify the apex of the triangle at the junction of the **anterior** and **posterior boundaries on the occiput**.
5. The roof is formed by the **cervical fascia** and partly by the lower part of the **platysma muscle**.
6. The floor is formed by **semispinalis capitis**, **splenius capitis**, **levator scapulae**, **scalenus medius** and **scalenus posterior**.
7. **Note the position of the cervical plexus, brachial plexus, subclavian artery, external jugular vein and accessory nerve.**

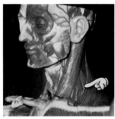
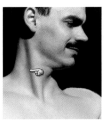

A B

202. ANTERIOR TRIANGLE OF THE NECK

1. Draw a vertical line in the median plane from the chin to the **suprasternal notch** on the **manubrium**. This line represents the **anterior border of the anterior triangle of the neck**.
2. Ask the model to fully rotate the **cervical spine** to the left.
3. Identify and palpate the right **sternocleidomastoid muscle** and mark the anterior border which represents the **posterior boundary of the anterior triangle of the neck**.
4. Palpate and surface mark the **inferior subcutaneous border of the ramus of the mandible** from the **chin** to the **angle of the mandible**.
5. This line represents the base of the **anterior triangle of the neck**.
6. The apex of the **anterior triangle** is formed by the junction of the **anterior** and **posterior borders**.

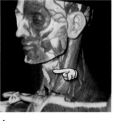
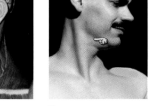

A B

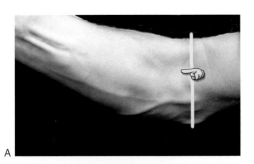

A

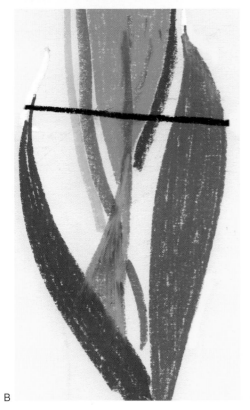

B

203. CUBITAL FOSSA

1. Draw a line across the anterior aspect of the **elbow** to connect the medial and lateral **epicondyles** of the **humerus** to represent the base of the **cubital fossa**.
2. The medial boundary is represented by a line drawn along the projected **lateral border of pronator teres**.
3. The lateral boundary is represented by a line drawn along the projected **medial border of brachioradialis**.
4. **Note how the tendon of biceps brachii subdivides the cubital fossa; note also the position of the radial and median nerves and brachial artery.**

204. POPLITEAL SPACE

1. Surface mark the **tendons of semimembranosus** and **semitendinosus** forming the upper and medial boundaries of the diamond-shaped **popliteal space.**
2. Surface mark the **tendon of biceps femoris** forming the upper and lateral boundaries of the **popliteal space**.
3. Surface mark the lateral border of the **medial head of gastrocnemius** forming the medial boundary.
4. Surface mark the medial border of the **lateral head of gastrocnemius** forming the lateral boundary.
5. **Note the position of the popliteal artery and vein, tibial and common peroneal nerves, short saphenous vein and lymph nodes in the popliteal fossa.**

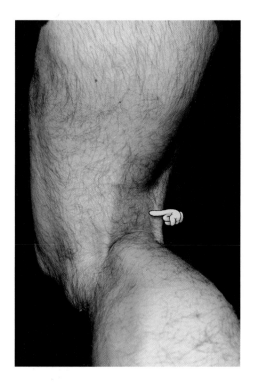

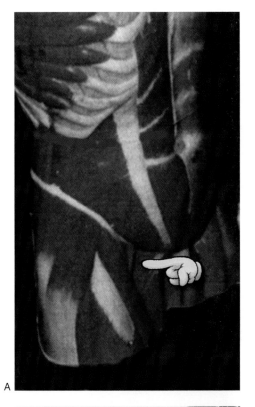

A

205. FEMORAL TRIANGLE

1. The base of the **femoral triangle** is formed by the **inferior edge of the inguinal ligament**, the lower border of the **external abdominal oblique muscle**.
2. Ask the model to flex, abduct and laterally rotate the **hip joint** against maximal resistance to demonstrate the **contour of sartorius**.
3. Maintaining the position, place resistance against the medial aspect of the **thigh** to demonstrate the **tendon** and **contour of adductor longus**.
4. The medial boundary of the **femoral triangle** is formed by the lateral border of **adductor longus**.
5. The lateral boundary of the **femoral triangle** is formed by the medial border of **sartorius**.
6. The apex of the **femoral triangle** is formed by the convergence of **sartorius** and **adductor longus**.
7. **Note the position of the femoral artery and vein, femoral nerve and lymph nodes in the femoral triangle.**

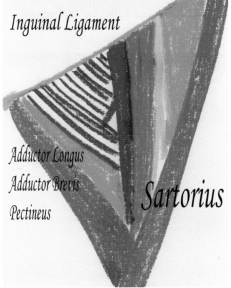

B

206. AXILLARY SPACE

1. Ask the model to abduct the **shoulder joint** to 90° to allow palpation of the muscles forming the boundaries of the truncated pyramidal-shaped **axillary space**.
2. Demonstrate against maximal resistance the action of **pectoralis major** and **minor** which form the anterior wall of **the axillary space** and surface mark the contour of **pectoralis major**.
3. Demonstrate against maximal resistance the action of **subscapularis, latissimus dorsi** and **teres major** which form the posterior wall of the **axillary space** and surface mark the contours of **latissimus dorsi** and **teres major**.
4. Demonstrate against maximal resistance the action of **serratus anterior** and note attachment to the ribs. Mark the position of the bodies of **ribs 1–6** and their respective **intercostal spaces**. These structures and upper fibres of **serratus anterior** form the medial wall of the **axillary space**.
5. Demonstrate against maximal resistance the contraction of **coracobrachialis** as it passes to its distal attachment on the medial surface of the **shaft of humerus**. Palpate and mark the upper one-third of the medial surface of the **shaft of humerus** which with **coracobrachialis** forms the lateral wall of the **axillary space**.
6. **Note that the truncated apex of the axillary space is directed upwards towards the root of the neck.**
7. **Note that the base of the axillary space is formed of fascia and skin which faces downwards.**

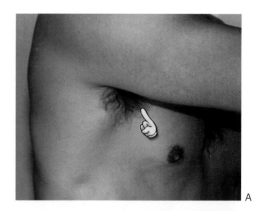

A

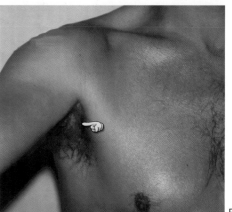

B

207. ANATOMICAL SNUFFBOX

1. Ask the model to fully extend the joints of the **thumb**.
2. Identify and surface mark the **tendon of extensor pollicis longus** as it passes to its distal attachment on the base of the **distal phalanx of the thumb**. This tendon forms the posterior boundary of the **anatomical snuffbox**.
3. Identify and surface mark the **tendon of extensor pollicis brevis** as it passes to its distal attachment on the base of the **proximal phalanx of the thumb**. This tendon forms the anterior boundary of the **anatomical snuffbox**.
4. **Note the floor of the anatomical snuffbox and location of the styloid process of radius, scaphoid, trapezium and base of the 1st metacarpal bone.**
5. **By abducting the thumb, identify and surface mark the tendon of abductor pollicis longus as it passes to its distal attachment to the base of the 1st metacarpal bone. This tendon can be observed and palpated anterior to the tendon of extensor pollicis brevis.**

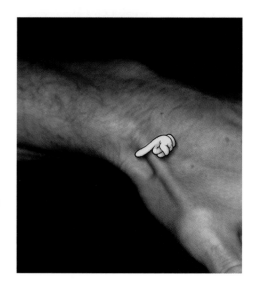

20

Deep Tendon Reflexes

208. C5 AND C6 BICEPS BRACHII

1. Place the model in sitting with the **right forearm** passively supported by the left hand of the examiner.
2. The thumb tip of the examiner's supporting hand should rest lightly on the **distal tendon attachment of the biceps brachii**.
3. Holding the percussion hammer firmly with the right hand, the examiner elicits a brisk contraction of the **muscle fibres of biceps brachii** by briskly tapping the **thumb** tip resting on the **tendon of biceps brachii**.
4. Alternatively the **tendon of biceps brachii** may be directly tapped but an improved response is usually obtained by tapping the examiner's fingertip which maintains a light pressure on the tendon, thus placing the muscle fibres on a slight stretch.

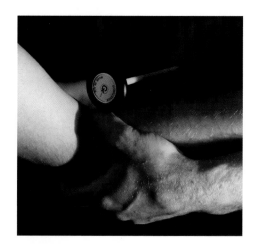

209. C5 AND C6 BRACHIORADIALIS

1. Place the model in sitting with the **right forearm** passively supported in the mid-prone position by the left hand of the examiner.
2. Holding the percussion hammer firmly with the right hand, the examiner elicits a brisk contraction of the **muscle fibres of brachioradialis** by briskly tapping the **distal extremity of the radius** immediately proximal to the **styloid process of radius** at the **distal attachment of the tendon of brachioradialis**.

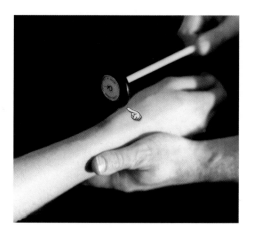

210. C6, C7 AND C8 TRICEPS BRACHII

1. Place the model in sitting, the **right arm** passively supported in abduction and medial rotation by the left hand of the examiner with the **elbow joint** of the model allowed to swing freely.
2. Holding the percussion hammer firmly with the right hand, the examiner elicits a brisk contraction of the **muscle fibres of triceps brachii** by tapping the **distal tendon** immediately proximal to its attachment to the superior aspect on the **olecranon process of ulna**.

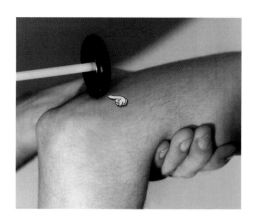

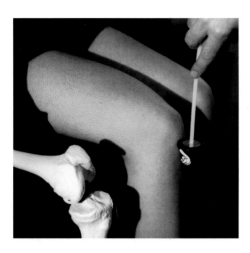

211. L2, L3 AND L4 QUADRICEPS FEMORIS

1. Place the model in high sitting with the **thighs** firmly supported and the **legs** hanging freely.
2. Holding the percussion hammer firmly, the examiner elicits a brisk contraction of the **quadriceps femoris muscle group** by tapping the **patellar tendon** immediately proximal to the superior bony border of the **tuberosity of tibia**.
3. Occasionally it may be necessary to request the model to perform the **'Jendrassk's' technique** of reinforcement to elicit a brisk response.

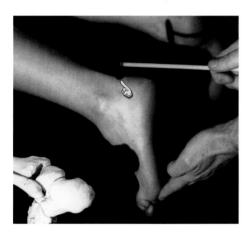

212. S1 AND S2 GASTROCNEMIUS AND SOLEUS

1. Ask the model to kneel comfortably supported on a chair with the **ankle** and **foot** hanging freely over the edge.
2. The fingertips of the examiner's left hand should be in firm contact against the **plantar surface** of the **foot** to be tested.
3. Holding the reflex percussion hammer in the right hand, the examiner elicits a brisk contraction of the superficial **calf muscles** by tapping the **achilles tendon** immediately proximal to its **distal attachment on the calcaneus**.

21

Dermatomes

213. Upper and lower limb
dermatomes

213. UPPER AND LOWER LIMB DERMATOMES

A dermatome may be defined as 'an area of skin supplied by one spinal nerve'.

Select one dermatome from the list below and surface mark the area of skin supplied by the spinal segment on a model in the anatomical position.

1. *C4 dermatome*: area of skin covering the **cervical** and **supraclavicular** areas extending to the medial and middle thirds of the **clavicle** and supraspinous area of the **scapula**.
2. *C5 dermatome*: area of skin covering the lateral third of the **clavicle**, **deltoid** and **biceps brachii**, lateral to the axial line of the **arm** and **forearm** over **palmaris longus** and **flexor carpi radialis**.
3. *C6 dermatome*: area of skin covering the upper fibres of **trapezius**, lateral area of **arm**, **elbow**, **forearm**, **thumb** and lateral aspect of **index finger**.
4. *C7 dermatome*: area of skin covering the **interscapular** posterior aspect of **shoulder**, **axilla**, **arm** and **forearm** and the anterior and posterior aspects of **index** and **middle fingers**.
5. *C8 dermatome*: area of skin covering the **interscapular**, **infraspinous** area of **scapula**, medial area of **arm**, **elbow** and **forearm** and the anterior and posterior areas of skin covering the **ring** and **little fingers**.
6. *T1 dermatome*: area of skin covering the lower **interscapular** area, inferior angle of **scapula**, medial aspect of **upper arm** and **axilla**, and anterior aspect of **arm** and **forearm**, immediately medial to the axial line proximal to the **wrist joint**.
7. *S5, S4, S3 and S2 dermatomes*: areas of skin, roughly circular covering the **perineum**, with **S5** in the centre, and **S4** and **S3** radiating outwards with **S2** forming a strip of skin supplying the posterior area of skin covering part of **gluteus maximus**, the **ischial tuberosity**, a strip of skin over the posterior midline of the **thigh**, **popliteal area** and **posterior leg** and medial aspect of the **calcaneus**.
8. *L1 dermatome*: a strip of skin sloping in a lateral direction from the level of the **12th thoracic vertebra**, **iliac crest**, anterior aspect of the **hip joint** towards the **pubis** and medial aspect of the upper **thigh**.
9. *L2 dermatome*: a strip of skin sloping in a lateral direction from the level of the **1st lumbar vertebra**, below the **iliac crest**, **gluteus medius**, anterior aspect of the upper one-third of the **thigh** and medially to the middle one-third of the **thigh**.
10. *L3 dermatome*: a strip of skin sloping in a lateral direction from the level of the **2nd lumbar vertebra**, below the **iliac crest**, above the **greater trochanter** and across the lateral, intermediate and medial aspects of the **thigh** to the medial aspect of the **knee joint** and upper medial aspect of the **leg**.
11. *L4 dermatome*: a strip of skin sloping in a lateral direction from the level of the **3rd lumbar vertebra**, below the **iliac crest**, the region of the **greater trochanter**, the lateral aspect of the **hip**, and down across the **patella**, anteromedial aspect of the **leg**, medial aspect of the **ankle** and **dorsum of foot** and the medial aspect of the **great toe**.

12. *L5 dermatome*: a strip of skin in the region of the **posterior superior iliac spine**, sloping in a lateral direction, over **gluteus maximus**, lateral aspect of **thigh** and **knee**, anterolateral aspect of **leg**, **2nd**, **3rd** and **4th toes** and the plantar aspect of **foot**.

13. *S1 dermatome*: a strip of skin in the region of the **posterior superior iliac spine**, sloping in a lateral direction over part of **gluteus maximus**, posterior aspect of **hip**, **ischial tuberosity**, **thigh** and **popliteal fossa**, lateral aspect of **ankle** and **5th toe** and plantar aspect of **foot**.

22

Myotomes

214. Myotomes

214. MYOTOMES

Select a **muscle** and demonstrate its action against maximal resistance to determine the integrity of **muscle function** and **spinal cord segments** supplying **motor neurones** to the **muscle** given a chart of the **muscle power assessment grades**. Manual resistance must be applied correctly to the leading surface of the moving limb to facilitate the correct functional pattern of movement, **e.g. latissimus dorsi, spinal cord segments C6, C7 and C8**.

CHART OF MUSCLE POWER ASSESSMENT GRADES

0 No muscle contraction evident

1 Flicker of muscle contraction

2 Active muscle contraction with effects of gravity counterbalanced

3 Active muscle contraction with movement through joint range against force of gravity

4 Active muscle contraction with movement through full joint range against gravity and application of maximal resistance against leading surface

5 Performs throughout full joint range demonstrating normal muscle group activity working as an agonist, antagonist, fixator or synergist in an everyday functional skilled movement against gravity and maximal resistance

SHOULDER GIRDLE, UPPER LIMB MUSCLES AND PRINCIPAL SPINAL CORD SEGMENTS OF ORIGIN

MUSCLE	SEGMENT(S)	TEST
Trapezius	C1–4	Place resistance against the **spine of scapula** and ask the model to elevate the **scapula**. Place resistance against the **vertebral border of scapula** and ask the model to retract the **scapula**.
Levator scapula	C3–5	Place resistance against the **base of the spine of scapula** and ask the model to elevate the **scapula**.
Rhomboids	C4–5	Place resistance against the **vertebral border of scapula** and ask the model to retract the **scapula**.
Supraspinatus	C4–5	Palpate the **supraspinous** area of **scapula**, place resistance against the lateral aspect of the **humerus** over the distal attachment of **deltoid** and ask the model to initiate abduction.
Infraspinatus	C4–6	Palpate the **infraspinous** area of **scapula**. Ask the model to flex the **elbow joint** to 90° and laterally rotate the **glenohumeral joint** against resistance applied to the **dorsum** of the **hand**.
Teres minor	C4–6	Palpate the upper lateral edge of the **axillary border** of **scapula**. Ask the model to flex the **elbow joint** to 90° and laterally rotate the **glenohumeral joint** against resistance applied to the **dorsum** of the **hand**.

MUSCLE	SEGMENT(S)	TEST
Subscapularis	C5–8	Palpate the **lesser tubercle** of the **humerus**. Ask the model to flex the **elbow joint** to 90° and medially rotate the **glenohumeral joint** against resistance applied to the **palm** of the **hand**.
Serratus anterior	C5–7	Palpate the **spine of scapula** and observe the **inferior angle**. Ask the model to place the fingertips on the clavicle and extend the **glenohumeral**, **elbow** and **wrist joints** against resistance applied to the **dorsum** of the **hand** in the action of punching forwards. The **inferior angle of scapula** is held against the **thoracic wall** as protraction takes place.
Teres major	C6–7	Palpate the inferior angle of **scapula** and the edge of the **axillary border**. Ask the model to flex the **elbow joint** to 90° and medially rotate the **glenohumeral joint** against resistance applied to the **palm**.
Deltoid	(C4) C5–6	Apply resistance to the lateral aspect of the lower one-third of the **shaft of humerus**. Ask the model to abduct the **glenohumeral joint** through a range from 15–90°. Palpate the anterior, middle and posterior fibres of **deltoid**.
Biceps brachii	C5–6	Apply resistance to the **palm** of the model. Ask the model to place the fingertips on the chin. Palpate **biceps brachii**.
Brachioradialis	C5–6	Ask the model to flex the **elbow joint** to 90° and place the **forearm** in a position of mid-pronation. Apply resistance to the lower one-third of **radius** and ask the model to flex the **elbow joint**.
Supinator	C5–6	Ask the model to flex the **elbow joint** to 90° and fully pronate the **palm**. Apply resistance to the **dorsum** of the **hand** and ask the model to supinate the **forearm**.
Pectoralis major	C5–8	*Clavicular head*: ask the model to abduct the **glenohumeral joint** to 120°. Apply resistance to the medial aspect of the **elbow joint**. Ask the model to adduct and flex the **glenohumeral joint**. Palpate the clavicular attachment of **pectoralis major**. *Sternal head*: ask the model to abduct the **glenohumeral joint** to 30°. Apply resistance to the medial aspect of the **elbow joint**. Palpate the sternal head of **pectoralis major**.
Extensor carpi radialis longus	C6–7	Apply resistance to the **dorsum** of the **hand**. Ask the model to fully extend and deviate the **wrist joint** towards the **radius**. Palpate **muscle belly** and **tendon**.
Pronator teres	C6–7	Ask the model to flex the **elbow joint** to 90° and place the **forearm** in full supination. Apply resistance to the **palm** of the **hand** and ask the model to pronate the **forearm**.

MUSCLE	SEGMENT(S)	TEST
Latissimus dorsi	C6–7–8	Palpate the inferior angle of **scapula**. Ask the model to cough. Palpate the muscle belly as it crosses the inferior angle of **scapula**. Ask the model to sit on a stool, grasp the stool, breathe out and lift the lower limbs and pelvis off the ground and stool.
Triceps	C6–7–8	Ask the model to place the fingertips on the **clavicle**. Apply resistance to the **dorsum** of the **hand**. Ask the model to fully extend the **elbow joint**.
Palmaris longus	C7–8–T1	Apply resistance to the tip of the **little finger** and **thumb**. Ask the model to flex the **wrist joint** and oppose the **little finger** and **thumb**. Identify the **tendon of palmaris longus** as it crosses the anterior surface of the **wrist joint** in the midline.
Flexor carpi radialis	C7–8	Apply resistance to the **thenar eminence**. Ask the model to flex and deviate the **wrist** towards the **radius**.
Extensor pollicis longus	C7–8	Apply resistance to the extensor surface of the terminal phalanx of the **thumb**. Ask the model to extend the **carpometacarpal joint** parallel to the plane of the **palm**.
Extensor pollicis brevis	C7–8	Apply resistance to the extensor surface of the proximal phalanx of the **thumb**. Ask the model to extend the **metacarpophalangeal joint** of the **thumb** parallel to the plane of the **palm**.
Abductor pollicis longus	C7–8	Apply resistance to the anterior surface of the proximal phalanx of the **thumb**. Ask the model to abduct the **carpometacarpal joint** of the **thumb** at a right angle to the plane of the **palm**.
Extensor carpi ulnaris	C7–8	Apply resistance to the **dorsum** and **ulnar** surface of the **hand**. Ask the model to extend the **radiocarpal joint** and deviate the hand in the direction of the **ulna**.
Extensor digitorum	C7–8	Ask the model to make a lightly clenched fist. Apply resistance to the **phalanges of the fingers** and **dorsum** of the **hand**. Ask the model to extend the **radiocarpal joint** and **metacarpophalangeal joints**.
Flexor carpi radialis	C6–7	Apply resistance to the anterior surface of the **thenar eminence**. Ask the model to flex the **radiocarpal joint** and deviate the **hand** towards the **radius**.
Flexor digitorum superficialis	C7–8–T1	Fix the position of the **proximal phalanx** of a **finger**. Apply resistance to the flexor surface of the **middle phalanx** of the **finger**. Ask the model to flex the **proximal interphalangeal joint** of the fixed **finger**.

MUSCLE	SEGMENT(S)	TEST
Flexor digitorum profundus	C7–8	Fix the position of the **middle phalanx** of a **finger** (index). Apply resistance to the flexor surface of the **terminal phalanx** of the **finger**. Ask the model to flex the **distal interphalangeal joint** of the finger.
Flexor pollicis longus	C7–8	Apply resistance to the **flexor surface** of the **distal phalanx** of the **thumb**. Ask the model to flex the **interphalangeal joint** of the **thumb**.
Abductor pollicis brevis	C8–T1	Apply resistance to the anterior surface of the **proximal phalanx** of the **thumb**. Ask the model to abduct the **carpometacarpal joint** at a right angle to the plane of the **palm**.
Flexor pollicis brevis	C8–T1	Fix the **proximal phalanx** of the **thumb**. Apply resistance to the flexor surface of the **proximal phalanx** of the **thumb**. Ask the model to flex the **interphalangeal joint** of the **thumb**.
Opponens pollicis	C8–T1	Apply resistance between the tip of the **distal phalanx** of the **little finger** and the tip of the **distal phalanx** of the **thumb**. Ask the model to oppose the tip of the **thumb** and the tip of the **little finger**.
Interossei and lumbricals	C8–T1	Ask the model to flex the **metacarpophalangeal joints** of the **fingers**. Ask the model to extend the **proximal interphalangeal joints** of the **fingers**. Apply resistance as the model extends the **proximal interphalangeal joints** as in the upstroke of writing or the action of smoothing a tablecloth.
Flexor carpi ulnaris	C7–8–T1	Apply resistance against the medial surface of the **little finger**. Ask the model to abduct the **little finger**, flex the **radiocarpal joint** and deviate the **hand** towards the **ulna**.
Abductor digiti minimi	C8–T1	Apply resistance to the medial surface of the **proximal phalanx** of the **little finger**. Ask the model to abduct the **little finger** in a medial direction away from the midline of the **hand**.
Flexor digiti minimi	C8–T1	Apply resistance to the flexor surface of the **proximal phalanx** of the **little finger**. Ask the model to flex the **metacarpophalangeal joint** of the **little finger**. Restrict movement of the **interphalangeal joints** to a position of **extension**.
Adductor pollicis	C8–T1	Apply resistance to the adductor surface of the **distal phalanx** of the **thumb**. Ask the model to adduct the **thumb** at a right angle to the plane of the **palm**.

PELVIC GIRDLE, LOWER LIMB MUSCLES AND PRINCIPAL SPINAL CORD SEGMENTS OF ORIGIN

MUSCLE	SEGMENT(S)	TEST
Iliopsoas	L1, 2 and 3	1. Place the model in lying with one **hip** and **knee** supported and flexed to a right angle and the **lumbar spine** supported. 2. Apply resistance to the anterior surface of the **thigh**. 3. Ask the model to flex the **hip joint** against resistance and palpate the **tendon of iliopsoas** as it passes over the anterior surface of the **hip joint** to its distal attachment on the **lesser trochanter**.
Quadriceps femoris	L2, L3 and L4	1. Place the model in sitting with the **hip** and **knee joints** flexed at a right angle. 2. Apply resistance to the anterior surface of the **shaft of tibia**. 3. Ask the model to fully extend the **knee joint** against resistance. 4. Palpate **vastus medialis, vastus lateralis** and **rectus femoris**.
Adductors (adductor magnus, longus and brevis, pectineus and gracilis)	L2, L3 and L4	1. Place the model in lying with one **hip joint** abducted to 30°. 2. Apply resistance to the medial surface of the **thigh** proximal to the **adductor tubercle**. 3. Ask the model to adduct the **hip joint** to the midline against resistance. 4. Palpate **adductor magnus**, **adductor longus** and **gracilis** on the medial aspect of the **thigh** proximal to the **adductor tubercle**.
Gluteus medius	L4, L5 and S1	1. Place the model in prone lying with the **hip joint** extended and the **knee joint** flexed to 90° and supported. 2. Apply resistance to the lateral surface of the supported **leg**. 3. Ask the model to rotate the **hip joint** in a medial direction against resistance. 4. Note the action of **gluteus medius** acting with **quadratus lumborum** in maintaining the level of the **iliac crest** during walking. 5. Palpate above the **greater trochanter** in the direction of the **anterior superior iliac spine** on the lateral aspect of the **ilium**.
Gluteus maximus	L5, S1 and S2	1. Place the model in prone lying with one **hip joint** extended and the **knee joint** flexed to 90° and supported. 2. Apply resistance to the posterior aspect of the **thigh** proximal to the **popliteal space**. 3. Ask the model to extend the **hip joint** against resistance while maintaining the **knee joint** flexed at 90°. 4. Palpate **gluteus maximus** as it passes over the **ischial tuberosity** towards its attachment on the **femur**.

MUSCLE	SEGMENT(S)	TEST
Semitendinosus, semimembranosus and biceps femoris	L5, S1 and S2	1. Place the model in **prone lying**. 2. Apply resistance to the posterior aspect of the **lower leg**. 3. Ask the model to flex the **knee joint** to 90° against resistance to demonstrate group action. 4. Ask the model to rotate the **knee joint** in a lateral direction to reinforce the action of **biceps femoris**. 5. Ask the model to rotate the **knee joint** in a medial direction to reinforce the action of **semitendinosus** and **semimembranosus**. 6. Palpate **semitendinosus** as it passes to the **medial tibial condyle**. 7. Palpate **biceps femoris** as it passes to its principal attachment on the **head of fibula**.
Soleus	Soleus	1. Ask the model to place one foot on a stool, **heel** over the edge, **ankle joint** in dorsiflexion and the **knee joint** flexed. 2. Apply resistance to the anterior aspect of the **thigh** proximal to the knee joint. 3. Ask the model to strongly plantarflex the **ankle joint** against resistance. 4. Palpate the lateral borders of **soleus** anterior to **gastrocnemius**.
Gastrocnemius	S1 and S2	1. Place the model in standing. 2. Ask the model to plantarflex the **ankle joints** and raise the **heels** against gravity. 3. Palpate **gastrocnemius** inferior to the **popliteal space**.
Tibialis posterior	L4 and L5	1. Place the model in a sitting position. 2. Apply resistance to the medial aspect and **dorsum** of the **foot** over the **tuberosity of navicular**. 3. Ask the model to plantarflex the **ankle joint** and invert the **foot** at the **subtalar** and **mid-tarsal joints** against resistance. 4. Palpate the tendon as it passes posterior to the **medial malleolus**, above **sustentaculum tali** towards the **tuberosity of navicular**.
Flexor digitorum longus	L5, S1 and S2	1. Place the model in a sitting position. 2. Apply resistance to the plantar surface of the **distal phalanx** of the **hallux**. 3. Ask the model to flex the **interphalangeal joint** of the **hallux** against resistance. 4. Palpate the tendons as they pass on the plantar aspect of the **foot** to the **lateral four distal phalanges**.
Tibialis anterior	L4 and L5	1. Place the model in a sitting position. 2. Apply resistance to the medial aspect and **dorsum** of the **foot** over the **medial cuneiform**. 3. Ask the model to dorsiflex the **ankle joint** and invert the **foot** at the **subtalar** and **mid-tarsal joints** against resistance. 4. Palpate the tendon passing over the medial aspect of the **foot** towards the **medial cuneiform** and base of the **1st metatarsal**.

MUSCLE	SEGMENT(S)	TEST
Extensor hallucis longus	L5 and S1	1. Place the model in a sitting position. 2. Apply resistance to the dorsal surface of the **distal phalanx** of the **hallux**. 3. Ask the model to extend the **interphalangeal joint** of the **hallux** against resistance. 4. Palpate the tendon passing lateral to **extensor hallucis longus** towards the **distal phalanx** of the **hallux**.
Extensor digitorum longus	L5 and S1	1. Place the model in a sitting position. 2. Apply resistance to the dorsal surface of the **distal phalanges** of the **lateral four toes**. 3. Ask the model to extend the **interphalangeal joints** of the **lateral four toes** against resistance. 4. Palpate the tendons passing to the **distal phalanges** of the **lateral four toes**.
Extensor digitorum brevis	L5 and S1	1. Place the model in a sitting position. 2. Apply resistance to the dorsal surface of the **lateral four toes**. 3. Ask the model to dorsiflex the **metatarsophalangeal joints** of the **lateral four toes** against resistance. 4. Palpate the muscle belly on the dorsum of the **foot** distal to the **lateral malleolus**.
Peroneus brevis	L5 and S1	1. Place the model in a sitting position. 2. Apply resistance to the lateral aspect of the dorsum of the **foot** over the base of the **5th metatarsal**. 3. Ask the model to evert the **subtalar** and **mid-tarsal joints** and lift the lateral border of the **foot**. 4. Palpate the tendon passing to the base of the **5th metatarsal** of the **foot**.
Peroneus longus	L5 and S1	1. Place the model in a sitting position. 2. Apply resistance to the lateral aspect of the dorsum of the **foot** over the **cuboid**. 3. Ask the model to evert the **subtalar** and **mid-tarsal joints**, lift the lateral border of the **foot** and draw up the medial longitudinal arch. 4. Palpate the tendon passing round the **lateral malleolus** of the **foot** towards the groove on the undersurface of the **cuboid**.

23

Lymphatics

215. LYMPH NODES OF THE FACE

1. Palpate the **infraorbital margin** and place one 2 mm circle inferior to the margin.
2. Mark two similar circles in the centre of the cheek muscle (**buccinator**).
3. Mark two circles immediately inferior to the **parotid duct**.
4. Mark three 2 mm circles on the anterior border of the **masseter muscle**.
5. Surface mark the **parotid gland** and mark small circles within the outline.
6. The efferent vessels of the superficial and deep **parotid lymph nodes** terminate in the **deep cervical chain**.

216. OCCIPITAL AND MASTOID LYMPH NODES

1. Surface mark the **mastoid process** and attachment of the **sternocleidomastoid** muscle.
2. Mark small circles to indicate the **lymph nodes** over the **mastoid** attachment of **sternocleidomastoid**.
3. Efferents drain into the upper group of the deep cervical chain of **lymph nodes**.

217. SUPERFICIAL CERVICAL LYMPH NODES

1. Surface mark the position of the **external jugular vein**.
2. Surface mark the outline of the **sternocleidomastoid muscle**.
3. Mark four or five small circles on or near to the **external jugular vein** as it lies on the **sternocleidomastoid muscle**.
4. Efferents drain into the **deep cervical lymph nodes**.

218. SUBMENTAL AND SUBMANDIBULAR LYMPH NODES

1. Ask the model to extend the **cervical spine** and surface mark the submental triangle.
2. Mark small circles within the triangle on the **mylohyoid** muscle.
3. Efferents drain into the **submandibular** group of **lymph nodes**.
4. Surface mark the **submandibular salivary gland**.
5. Draw a number of small circles on the surface of the **submandibular salivary gland** to represent the **submandibular lymph nodes**.
6. Efferents drain into the **deep cervical chain of lymph nodes**.

219. DEEP CERVICAL LYMPH NODES

1. Identify the contour of **sternocleidomastoid** by asking the model to rotate the **cervical spine** to place the chin close to the **acromion process** of the opposite shoulder. Surface mark.
2. Draw a line from the **occipital bone** to the supraclavicular triangle of the neck following the contour of **sternocleidomastoid**.
3. Surface mark the position of the **internal jugular vein**.
4. The **deep cervical lymph nodes** are made up of a superior and inferior group deep to **sternocleidomastoid** and may be surface marked by grouping small circles along the surface marking of the **sternocleidomastoid muscle** and **internal jugular vein**.
5. Efferents drain into the **thoracic duct** or the **right lymphatic duct**.

220. FIVE GROUPS OF AXILLARY LYMPH NODES

1. Ask the model to place the upper limb in a position of abduction and lateral rotation.
2. Surface mark the **axillary vein**, **pectoralis minor** and the boundaries of the **axillary space**.
3. Draw 2 mm circles along the medial aspect of the **axillary vein** to represent the **lateral group of lymph nodes** draining the **upper extremity**.
4. Draw 2 mm circles along the inferior border of **pectoralis minor** to represent the **pectoral group of lymph nodes** draining the lateral area of the breast and from the anterior and lateral areas above the **umbilicus**.
5. Draw 2 mm circles along the posterior boundary of the **axillary space** to represent the **subscapular group of lymph nodes** adjacent to the **subscapular blood vessels**. This group drains the dorsal aspect of the **trunk**.
6. Draw 2 mm circles in the **base of the axilla** to represent the **central group of lymph nodes** draining the **pectoral** and **subscapular** groups.
7. Mark the apex of the **coracoid process** and projected outline of **pectoralis minor**. The **apical group of lymph nodes** lies deep to the muscle belly of **pectoralis minor**. Efferent vessels form the **subclavian trunk** which passes to the **thoracic duct** or **right lymphatic duct**.

221. LYMPH NODES OF THE LOWER LIMB

Part 1

1. Surface mark the position of the **short saphenous vein** in the **popliteal space**.
2. Identify the pulse of the **popliteal artery**.
3. Mark a 2 mm circle to indicate a lymph node adjacent to the pulse of the **popliteal artery**.
4. Mark four 2 mm circles to indicate lymph nodes close to the termination of the **short saphenous vein** in the **popliteal space**.

Part 2

1. Draw a gently curving convex line to indicate the **inguinal ligament** from the **anterior superior iliac spine** towards the **symphysis pubis**.
2. Surface mark the termination of the **long (great) saphenous vein**.
3. Draw a short line of 2 mm circles inferior to the **inguinal ligament** to indicate the position of the **superficial inguinal group of lymph nodes**.
4. Surface mark the position of the **femoral vein** medial to the pulse of the **femoral artery**.
5. Draw 2 mm circles medial to the **femoral vein** close to the termination of the **long (great) saphenous vein**.

24

Miscellaneous

222. OPENING OF THE VERIFORM APPENDIX INTO THE CAECUM

1. Draw a vertical line on the **abdomen** to represent the **right lateral vertical plane**.
2. Draw a horizontal line on the **abdomen** to represent the **intertubercular plane**.
3. Mark the junction of the **right lateral vertical plane** where it crosses the **intertubercular plane**.
4. The opening of the **appendix** into the **caecum** is positioned inferior and medial to the junction of the two planes.

223. ASCENDING, TRANSVERSE AND DESCENDING COLON ON THE ABDOMEN

1. Mark the intertubercular plane, right and left lateral vertical planes and **right 9th costal cartilage**.
2. Draw a line upwards from the intertubercular plane, just lateral to the lateral vertical plane to the **right 9th costal cartilage** to represent the **ascending colon** to the point where the **colon** turns to form the **hepatic flexure**.
3. Draw a line from the **right 9th costal cartilage** crossing the midline at the level of the **2nd lumbar vertebra** to the **left 8th costal cartilage** where the **transverse colon** forms the **splenic flexure**.
4. Draw a line from the **8th costal cartilage** passing downwards just lateral to the left lateral vertical plane to the level of the posterior part of the **iliac crest** to represent the **descending colon**.

224. COURSE OF THE EXTERNAL JUGULAR VEIN

1. Ask the model to demonstrate the left **sternocleidomastoid muscle** by rotating the **cervical spine** to the right.
2. Palpate and mark the left **angle of mandible**.
3. Mark a point immediately superior to the midpoint of the **shaft of clavicle**.
4. Mark the course of the **external jugular vein** from where it commences just posterior to the **angle of mandible**, passes downwards towards the midpoint of the **shaft of clavicle**. At this point the vein pierces deep fascia to join the **subclavian vein**.

225. COURSE OF THE INTERNAL JUGULAR VEIN

1. Take the pulse of the **common carotid artery** and mark the location.
2. Take the pulse of the **internal carotid artery** and mark the location.
3. Draw a line from the **lobule of the ear** to a point between the sternal and clavicular attachments of **sternocleidomastoid**, parallel and lateral to the course of the **internal** and **common carotid arteries** to indicate the course of the **internal jugular vein**.

226. COURSE OF THE TWO URETERS ON THE POSTERIOR ASPECT OF THE TRUNK

1. Draw a horizontal line to represent the transpyloric plane crossing the **1st lumbar vertebra**.
2. Identify the spinous process of the **2nd lumbar vertebra**.
3. Draw two parallel lines, each 3 cm from the midline, commencing level with the spinous process of the **2nd lumbar vertebra** passing downwards for 25 cm to a point level with the **posterior superior iliac spines** where the right and left **ureters** enter the **bladder**.

Appendix –
Notes on
Terminology

NAMING STRUCTURES

Examples of how equivalent structures can be named from English, Latin or Greek:

ENGLISH	LATIN	GREEK
Chin	Mental	Genial
Bone like a little boat	Navicular	Scaphoid
Cheek bone	Malar	Zygoma
Collar bone	Clavicle	Cleido
Brooch pin	Fibular	Peroneal
Wall	Parietal	Somatic
Internal organ	Visceral	Splanchnic
The arm and shoulder	Brachium	Omos
Finger bones	Digits	Phalanges

EXAMPLES OF SKELETAL MUSCLE NAMES

Skeletal muscles may have names related to their **function**, **position** or **shape**. Others have combined names (e.g. serratus anterior or palmaris longus).

Function
Flexor carpi radialis, levator scapulae, erector spinae, extensor indices, levator anguli oris, supinator, pronator teres, abductor digiti minimi, corrugator, extensor digitorum brevis, opponens pollicis.

Position
Brachialis, coracobrachialis, tibialis posterior, infraspinatus, peroneus brevis, supraspinatus, tibialis anterior, interossei, subscapularis.

Shape
Quadriceps, triceps, deltoid, trapezius, semitendinosus, piriformis, gracilis, rhomboid major, teres minor, soleus, gastrocnemius, lumbricals.

APPLYING TERMINOLOGY

All anatomical terminology is defined with a model in the anatomical position, the body in the upright standing position, palms facing forward. Terminology remains constant whatever the position taken up by the model.
- Structures nearer to the head (cranial) are **superior**, those closer to the tail end (caudal) are **inferior**.
- The **anterior surface** of the hand facing forwards is known as the **palmar surface**.
- The **posterior surface** facing backwards is known as the **dorsal surface**.
- The **dorsal area** may also be known as the **dorsum** (as in the *dorsum of the foot*).
- A plane **parallel to the anterior surface** is known as a **coronal plane**.

- A plane at **right angles to the coronal plane** is termed the **sagittal plane**.
- A plane through the **midline of the body** is called the **median plane**.
- Structures **near to the midline** of the body are **medial to the midline** and those structures **farther away from the midline** are said to be **lateral to the midline**.
- The **thumb** is placed on the **lateral side of the hand**.
- The **big toe** is placed on the **medial side of the foot**.
- **Distance** from a feature is indicated by the words **proximal** and **distal**.
- A feature placed **proximal** may be defined as being **nearer** to and **distal** as being **farther away** from a given point.
- **Superficial** and **deep** are used to describe **depth of structures** related to the surface of the skin.
- The movement of **flexion** takes place when the **anterior surfaces** are **brought together** (as in *flexion of the elbow joint*).
- **Adduction** takes place when the structures are moved **towards the midline**.
- **Abduction** is brought about when limbs are moved **away from the midline** of the trunk (as in raising the upper limbs to shoulder level).
- **Rotation** of the limbs can be medial or lateral **rotation** taking place at the **glenohumeral joint** or **hip joint**.
- **Pronation** and **supination** occur when the **radius is rotated** in respect to the position of the ulna.
- **Inversion** and **eversion** take place in the **tarsal joints of the foot**.
- The **pre-axial surface** or border of a limb is the **nearest border to the head**.
- The **post-axial surface** or border of a limb is the nearest border to the **tail end of the body**.

Glossary of Anatomical Terms

This is a simple glossary of anatomical terms designed around the topics covered in the sections. These have been taken from a list of about 5000 terms approved in 1895 and revised in 1950. Each part has one name, which should be as short and simple as possible. Related terms should be similar (e.g. radial artery and radial nerve).

Abduction to move away (Latin *ab* = from, *ducere* = to lead)
Adduction to move towards (Latin *ad* = towards)
Acetabulum vinegar cup (Latin *acetum* = vinegar)
Acromion point of the shoulder (Greek *akros* = point, *omos* = shoulder)
Anconeus related to the elbow (Greek *agkos* = bend of the arm)
Annular ring-shaped (Latin *annulus* = a ring)
Articular joint (Latin = *articulatus* = jointed)
Astragalus ankle bone (Greek) (Latin = *talus*)
Atlas Greek god Atlas who supported the earth
Axilla armpit (Latin)
Axis pivot (Latin)

Bursa sac (Greek)

Calcis of the heel (Latin *calcar* = a spur)
Capitulum small head (Latin *caput* = head)
Carotid (Greek *karos* = sleep)
Cartilage (Latin *cartilago* = cartilage)
Cervical (Latin *cervix* = neck)
Condyle (Greek *condulos* = knuckle)
Coronal (Latin *corona* = a crown)
Cricoid signet ring (Greek *cricos* = a ring, *eidos* = form)
Cruciate cross (Latin *crux* = a cross)
Cuneiform (Latin *cuneus* = wedge)
Diarthrosis movable joint (Greek *dia* = through, *arthron* = joint)

Digital (Latin = a finger)

Epi upon (Greek)

Femur thigh (Latin)
Fibula buckle (Latin)
Foramen opening (Latin)
Fovea pit (Latin)

Glenoid (Greek *glene* = cavity, *eidos* = form)

Hallux (Latin *hallex* = great toe)
Humerus arm bone (Latin)

Innominate no name (Latin *in* = not, *nomem* = a name)
Ischium (Greek *ischion* = hip)

Jugular (Latin *jugulum* = neck)

Labrum lip (Latin)
Lamina a plate (Latin)
Lumbar loins

Manubrium a handle (Latin)
Mastoid nipple-shaped (Greek *mastos* = breast, *eidos* = form)
Median midline
Metacarpa (Greek *meta* = after, *karpos* = wrist)

Nuchae (Latin = neck)

Obturator (Latin *obturare* = to seal, obturator foramen = sealed foramen)
Olecranon (Greek *olekranon* = point of the elbow)

Parietal wall of an organ (Latin *parietalis*)
Patella a plate (Latin)
Pelvis a basin (Latin)
Phalanges phalanx (Greek)
Pisiform (Latin *pisus* = a pea, *forma* = shape)
Pollex a thumb (Latin)

Radius a spoke (Latin)
Ramus a branch (Latin)

Sagittal straight (Latin *sagitta* = arrow)
Saphenous visible (Greek *saphenes* = manifest)
Scaphoid (Latin *scapha* = a skiff, Greek *skaphe*)
Scapula shoulder (Latin)
Sesamoid sesame seed (Greek)
Sternum (Greek *sternon* = the breast)
Sustentaculum support (Latin)
Suture seam (Latin)
Syndesmosis a joint where two bones are bound together by fibres (Greek = band)

Trochanter a raised bony protuberance (Greek *trochanter* = a runner)
Trochlea pulley (Latin)
Tuberosity a rounded smooth raised surface (Latin *tubersitas*)

Xiphoid (Greek *xiphos* = sword, *eidos* = shape)